Like Any Other Woman: The Lived Experience of Gynaecological Cancer

Jac Saorsa with Rebecca Phillips

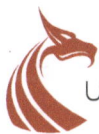

Cardiff University Press

Gwasg Prifysgol Caerdydd

Published by
Cardiff University Press
Cardiff University
PO Box 430
1st Floor, 30-36 Newport Road
Cardiff CF24 0DE
https://cardiffuniversitypress.org

First published 2019

Cover design by Hugh Griffiths

Front cover: *Diagnosis* (oil paint, chalk and pastel on canvas with oil ground.
Original artwork by Jac Saorsa)

Print and digital versions typeset by Siliconchips Services Ltd.

ISBN (Paperback): 978-1-911653-05-9
ISBN (PDF): 978-1-911653-08-0
ISBN (EPUB): 978-1-911653-06-6
ISBN (Kindle): 978-1-911653-07-3

DOI: https://doi.org/10.18573/book2

The full text of this book has been peer-reviewed to ensure high academic
standards. For full review policies, see https://www.cardiffuniversitypress.org/
site/research-integrity/

To read the free, open access version of this book online, visit
https://doi.org/10.18573/book2 or scan this QR code with your
mobile device:

Contents

Illustrations

Foreword

Like Any Other Woman is Becky's story of living through treatment and beyond for a gynaecological cancer and the profound impact that it has had on her life and that of her family. It takes courage to share the story of such a difficult journey and we, as readers, can learn much from it, but just possibly, and I hope it's true for Becky and the other women that have shared snippets of their cancer journeys, the very act of storytelling can be therapeutic in itself. Storytelling is a powerful way to convey experience and help the reader gain new insights from another's perspective. It teaches us to listen, to look past the facts, to hear and understand in our own way the real story, the real meaning of dis-ease.

Jac Saorsa helps us negotiate the stories and challenges us to question the history (her-story) of the disease in order to unearth, and maybe to begin to understand, the experience of the women themselves and the implications of a diagnosis of gynaecological malignancy. In the book, there are other stories that weave in and out of those of the main protagonists, including those of Jac herself, the surgeons, the medical and nursing staff, the mother, the husband. We can all learn from these stories and in so doing aspire to making the journeys just a little easier, whether that be as a healthcare professional, a family member or a friend. Each of us will take away different messages, but the central importance of supportive partners and the families to those affected will be evident to all. As a mother, daughter, friend, sister, wife, doctor and cancer surgeon myself, there are many aspects of *Like Any Other Woman* that resonate with my own experience, living alongside those journeying with illness.

Gynaecological disease is often shrouded in stigma, embarrassment and discomfort. There is often ignorance, and sometimes shame. In cases of gynaecological cancer these attributes may be heightened, the afflicted 'patient' feeling isolated and alone while facing an uncertain future.

One of the early things I appreciated in the book was the importance of a 'diagnosis' or naming the unknown, classifying the disease and perhaps making one feel more in control. The disease process hasn't changed, but naming it offers hope that now it is known something 'can be done', that somehow it makes sense. One of the women puts this very clearly in her own words. 'Actually it was massive relief, because there was one stage when I thought I was going mad – I can't think of another way to put it – a freak of nature, because nobody seemed to know what I was talking about.' Diagnosis often comes with 'relief' therefore, although, as a doctor, I can't help but feel this might sometimes be a cruel relief once the enormity of the treatment process comes into view. But still, in *Like Any Other Woman*, even finding the 'VIN clinic' sign was associated with relief, the disease was named, known, classified.

The manner in which any cancer diagnosis is imparted cannot be underestimated in terms of impact on a patient and her (or his) family. The manner, the tone, the surroundings will be forever imprinted in the memory, even if little else is remembered after the fateful words are spoken. The diagnosis should be given with thoughtfulness, empathy, kindness and skill, no matter how 'together' a patient seems. It saddens me therefore that empathy is sometimes lacking, and the harsh surroundings of many hospital wards, clinics and even quiet rooms are rarely conducive to the giving of bad news. The skills for the task include acknowledging the pain and fear of a cancer diagnosis and seeing the person, the family, the friends, beyond the words of a diagnosis and all members of a healthcare team, from the most senior to the junior, have their part to play. The smallest acts of kindness can make the journey more tolerable.

One quandary for a surgeon performing an operation to remove a malignant tumour is 'how much to cut away'. It is a fine balancing act between removing a cancer in its entirety, and thereby reducing the chance of recurrence, and potentially causing long-term morbidity and disability from the removal of tissue and disruption of normal anatomy and function. The old adage of a surgeon that 'cold steel cures' has to be weighed against the ultimate cost for the patient. In *Like Any Other Woman*, Jac Saorsa reflects on the violence of surgery, but the doctor is doing battle against tissue that is 'out of control', 'malignant' and the margins between cure and harm may be narrow or even overlap. Surgery is an art, by nature unnatural and therefore somewhat violent, but with an entirely different motive to true violence, where attack or injury is done with malevolent intent. One does need to understand the intent of surgery, 'radical' versus 'palliative', where radical is to effect a cure and palliative is to relieve symptoms for varying amounts of time. Radical surgery also has to be weighed against preservation of function and limitation of morbidity.

Jac Saorsa also notes the surgeon works with 'dominance'. I would suggest a better word might perhaps be 'determination'. The surgeon has to commence, continue and conclude the operation, hopefully removing the tumour and halting the progression of malignancy. The surgeon has to be focused, has to be in control of her team, her operative field. In a resource-limited health service a surgeon may well be concerned that an operation is completed on time, otherwise the patient following next on the operating list may be cancelled, and who knows when she can next be fitted in? Who knows what lengths she and her family have gone to in getting her to the hospital that day – time off work, childcare sorted, goodbyes said, travel arrangements made? The responsibility to get through an operating list rests heavily on a surgeon's shoulders.

A subtheme running alongside the stories in *Like Any Other Woman* is that of informed consent. It highlights questions that are always pertinent, and in many ways unanswerable. How far are these patients informed? Did they have the information to make the decision to proceed with surgery? Did they understand the risks of morbidity or continuing disability? To what extent do these women have a choice anyway, informed or otherwise, to proceed or not in the face of potentially life-saving, but also life-changing, surgery? In the face of complex procedures with significant attendant risks of severe morbidity, is informed consent really ever achievable? Who determines what and how much information a woman needs to make an informed decision?

In Becky's case, where a hemi-vulvectomy became a radical vulvectomy, a low chance of colostomy became a high chance of colostomy, and a reversal of colostomy led to sustained severe pain, would more information have changed her mind or have informed her consent to proceed? In many cases I suspect patients 'consent' because they see that they have little or no alternative in the face of cancer. Choice and autonomy are given up in the hope that the cancer can be beaten or, at least, life extended. They 'have' to place their life in the doctor's hands. With hindsight the decision-making process may be easier but it's not a position we have at the outset. How many patients live with regret or rage against the loss of function and, in cases of gynaecological malignancy, loss of childbearing potential, loss of femininity? 'Was it worth it?' is not something we dare ask our patients and perhaps something we wouldn't dare ask ourselves if we were like any other woman. By the end of *Like Any Other Woman* I suspect Becky would say that it was worth it and certainly her courage to endure and hope is inspirational to all of us.

Alison Fiander
Gynaecological surgeon
January 2019

Word by word, the language of women so often begins with a whisper.

Terry Tempest Williams

Introduction

At 24 she was diagnosed with vulval cancer, an 'old ladies' disease', just four months before her wedding. She wrote it all down, her pain, her hopes, her fears. She asked me to edit her work but I could not: her writing is just too authentic not to be heard on its own terms, so we agreed that I would write a book in which I would express through words (both hers and mine) and imagery her experiences and the resonances with those of other women who have similar conditions. This is the book. It 'speaks the unspeakable' in a polyvocal form of language that everyone will understand, according to their uniquely subjective interpretation. It will help people appreciate what a cancer diagnosis can feel like, and how it can impact a life.

Like Any Other Woman has been written over three years, and in different places and different stages of both our lives, Becky's and mine. Things have changed and moved on for both of us but there has been an unbroken thread between us defined by text messages and mutual encouragement. Becky sent me her manuscript page by page, painstakingly beaten out on her small iPad. She copied it word for word from her handwritten notebooks and emailed it to me as attachments with the whole of a short message carried in the subject line. As I read now I am constantly taken back to the first time I met with her in the bare little room at the VIN (Vulval Intraepithelial Neoplasia) Clinic at Llandough Hospital in Cardiff. It was the spring of 2012.

The young woman I met then is, within these pages, being reconstructed in her own words, and her story provides the context for everything that she told me that day. It is a raw and deeply honest outpouring of how she has experienced and managed her life throughout a time when her illness has necessitated so many changes, both practically and emotionally, and I feel strangely humble as I pare it down into extracts that will together become the meaningful core of

How to cite this book chapter:
Saorsa, J. with Phillips, R. 2019. *Like Any Other Woman: The Lived Experience of Gynaecological Cancer.* Pp. 1–6. Cardiff: Cardiff University Press. DOI: https://doi.org/10.18573/book2.a. License: CC-BY-NC-ND 4.0

the present book. Chronologically narrated, it is more thoughtful and structurally coherent than the conversation that we had, but no less authentic for being so. Once more, and as she will again, Becky allows me to enter her world, and as I write I feel very deeply the responsibility and the obligation to respect the boundaries, to go where she leads and create only shallow footprints beside and between the ones she leaves.

The project

Becky was one of the first women to agree to be involved at the very beginning of the *Drawing Women's Cancer* project, and this book is as much celebration of her courage and resilience throughout her experiences of being diagnosed with and treated for vulval cancer at the tender age of 24 years as it is a creative commentary of the project as a whole. I have written *Like Any Other Woman*, therefore, not necessarily *for* Becky, whose personal story is the basis for what is set down here, nor even *with* her, as she has gifted me with her trust that I will use and edit her manuscript with the respect it deserves. I have written the book *because* of her, and because there is a need for all women who have walked in Becky's shoes to be heard.

Drawing Women's Cancer first took to the stage in the hospital theatre in early 2012. It began as a small pilot study carried out through a collaboration between myself, as the artist, and Dr T, former consultant surgeon in gynaecological oncology in Cardiff, in the UK. The initial study focused primarily on women suffering with vulval cancer, the most rare form of the five gynaecological cancers. It was intended to articulate the experience of illness through art and thereby raise awareness and increase general understanding of the condition through a public exhibition. The project involved my having informal and continuing conversations with patients over the period of their treatment, and with their carers and health professionals, and the transcripts of these encounters provided me with the basis for a creative and exploratory drawing process based on my experience of their experience.

Back then, when the original project was in its infancy, its true value and purpose remained nascent under a cloak of academic research, but it has grown, evolved. The cloak has now been cast aside and the project has gathered around itself instead so much support from so many different audiences who have responded in their own ways to its means of being. It should be noted therefore that, in the interest of integrity and with deep respect for all of the women who have worked with me, while I have maintained ethical boundaries, I have set aside any pretence of scientific detachment as the project continues to progress and develop.

Drawing Women's Cancer has since generated several further projects involving my working with patients and medical professionals in the UK, the USA and Africa, and all of these are fully documented on the websites listed in the references section of this book, but in relation to the ongoing original project, since that first study, I have worked with women with all forms of gynaecological cancer and breast cancer. The hybrid results, in public art exhibitions and in digital and written form, offer a form of meta-language that is created in and through each separate interpretation and becomes itself a 'voice', intended to communicate across the boundaries of convention and taboo and articulate the nuances of suffering. And so, at the time of writing this book in 2018, and even though the *Drawing Women's Cancer* project has indeed achieved some 'academic' success, it is its 'soul', the life force that keeps the work I do relevant and fundamentally subjective, that has endured. Now, following a deeper and more honest trajectory, the narrative that continues through *Like Any Other Woman* adopts a fractured, yet perhaps more realistic, character in the way that it interweaves empathic orientation to the suffering 'Other' with subjective understandings of time, place and meaning, and with the fundamental idea of the futility of process and expectation when trying to understand the illness experience.

The book

Like Any Other Woman draws on many voices. It is Bakhtin's heteroglossia, a 'hybrid utterance', a multilayered and richly textured fabric of womanhood wherein my own voice as author is interwoven with Becky's voice, as taken from transcripts of conversations between us and from her own reflective writings, and with the voices of other women who have felt the devastating impact of a cancer diagnosis. All of these women's experiences, both positive and negative, are fundamental to this book being written at all, and through working with them and getting to know them, albeit through mainly short and intensive encounters, I have come to understand, deeply, what the *Drawing Women's Cancer* project is really all about. Like the project as a whole, this book is more than a piece of academic research. It seeks to offer a profoundly 'human' exploration of the overall existential, or 'lived' experience of being treated for all forms of gynaecological cancer, experience which extends not only to the patient herself but to all those who love and care for her. As such, the names of the professional staff involved have been reduced to the initial letter in order to preserve a level of anonymity, while, as all the women who worked with me in the project gave their full consent, all their first names remain unchanged.

All artwork in this book is reproduced from original drawings made by the author Jac Saorsa for the *Drawing Women's Cancer* project. The image on the front cover is the 'signature piece' for the project as a whole. It was made directly from the author's experience of listening to a woman describing the shock of diagnosis, and the piece seeks to convey, through the multilayered image, the physical 'shuddering' and feeling of disassociation that the woman described.

A note on method

My approach to my work as a whole is derived from an autoethnographic perspective. It is an approach that legitimises the subjective personal context, and this means that I write from the basis of my own experience as artist, and most importantly as human being, about the experiences of the women I have worked with. Through talking with these women, and simply being with them in clinics, waiting rooms and sometimes their homes, in witnessing the surgical procedures they undergo and in being there for them in the aftermath, I temporarily inhabit their unique worlds. Moreover, in being so present, I am co-creating and co-habiting with each woman a separate world, a world 'in-between', a world where time itself takes on different dimensions and is transformed into multiple and differing forms of layered meaningful experience. This is the world wherein we both become subjects of a combined narrative that renders illusory and meaningless any idea of distance and objectivity.

Unlike conventional ethnography, *auto*ethnography values the concept of 'presence' in terms of authorship, given that there is no meaningful separation between the author (in this case myself) and my experience of the 'Other'. The autoethnographic approach therefore begins from the proposition that meaningful experience, and especially in terms of human relations, is defined by subjectivity, and where ethnographic writing is consistent with ethnographic experience, there is no way of separating my 'presence', within experience, from my authorship of it. Autoethnographic account is therefore a personal narrative that simultaneously draws upon and explores experience with a focus on subjective responses more than on theoretical or analytical critique, or on the beliefs or practices of others. It challenges both the meaningful authenticity of a standard research text, along with the idea that there can be any universally acceptable and finite 'truth' in terms of individual experience, and therefore cannot be judged by traditional positivist criteria. In *Like Any Other Woman*, I am using the autoethnographic approach in order to seek an alternative, narrative 'truth' through a showing rather than a telling. The words and images that derive from my encounters with women are not intended merely to represent their experiences, but to evoke them. Here, the autoethnographic approach defines both the method and the result.

But the personal narratives as set out in this book, in layered and juxtaposing accounts, along with the experimental, or non-academic, structure are not purely autobiographical. The prefix 'auto' is appended to ethnography, rather than to biography, for good reason. For the most part, *Like Any Other Woman* is written in the present tense and from my own perspective as artist and author. But time and subject shifts necessarily become integral to the nature of the book as, contextualised in a complex temporality, it remains true to Becky's chronological narrative, written in her own words, and distinguished from the rest of the text by being set in italics. Her spoken words, taken from digital recordings of our conversations, are quoted in the book as part of the general text. The book is true also to the narratives of other women involved in the *Drawing Women's*

Cancer project. Their words, also taken directly from transcripts made from digital recordings of our meetings, both reflect and relate to the main story. They become the 'sutures' that hold the separate parts of the text together.

It is important to note that the autoethnographic account acknowledges, and indeed values, the complex and inescapable link between the personal and the cultural. Autoethnography embraces vulnerability with empathy, and, methodologically, it narratively structures existential crises and experiences that impact on lives and alter fundamental levels of meaning. Moreover, it invites moral and ethical dialogue and it offers an alternative to static and binary relationships in a social context. According to Denzin, the guiding question for any autoethnographer is as follows:

> Have I created an experiential text that allows me (and you) to understand what I have studied and experienced, where such understanding occurs when you and I are able to interpret what has been described within a framework that is subjectively, emotionally and causally meaningful. (Denzin, 2014)

I must leave it to you, the reader of the rest of this book, to decide.

Ultimately, *Like Any Other Woman* speaks to the suffering that cancer causes, and to the profound human experience of renegotiating the physical and emotional balance between sickness and health when that balance is tipped by the onset of disease. But it is not a book about the cancer itself, the etiological world of causes and symptoms. Neither is it about the medical world of biomedical interventions that characterise individual treatment regimes. It is rather about what it feels like when all sense of normality, all the expectations of a future that accompany good health, suddenly become submerged in degrees of suffering that impact both on the individual and on the people who care for and about her.

> *It was around 2007 when things starting getting a bit difficult in the bedroom department. I just didn't want to have sex because it was too painful and the situation would always cause an argument between us. I tried to explain, but I don't think Matthew understood how painful it was for me. I think he thought it was him, but it certainly wasn't and I didn't want him thinking there was something wrong. A lot of women would agree with me that sitting a man down and trying to explain things like that is not easy at all and after the arguments I thought, 'Right I'm going to have to get this sorted', so I booked an appointment to see a doctor about my problem. I was worried about how I was going to explain things to the doctor but in the few days I was waiting for my appointment I found a lump in my groin area and I noticed my skin underneath had starting turning like a black colour. I thought to myself, 'I'm glad I have made an appointment now.'*

Becky began writing soon after the first exhibition for the *Drawing Women's Cancer* project at the Senedd Welsh Assembly building in Cardiff. On the opening night, when foul weather brought enough rain to flood the whole of Cardiff Bay, Becky lit up the room with her smile and I watched with awe as this incredible woman, who sees herself as 'quite a shy person really', sat talking freely and openly with politicians and doctors about everything that she had been through. Neither of us knew then how much more was to come. How much more her body would have to endure and how her heart was destined to ache almost to breaking. Her words, written down, belie the life force that is behind them, the same life force that has sustained her over the years through the grief over several deaths in her family and over the loss of her own health. For me, her writing is raw and genuine, without guile. It goes beyond simply a chronological narration of events and provides a true insight into Becky's character. For me, her story is written both in and between the lines.

A major part of the context of Becky's writing is encapsulated in an important fact that I am acutely aware of. She wants very much for me to emphasise her enduring and deeply loving relationship with Matthew, her husband. In many ways, for Becky at least, the story is as much Matthew's as it is hers. It is Matthew who she has turned to throughout, and it is only Matthew who knows her for everything that she is. In a recent text she sent me she is emphatic:

> I would like you to bring everything in that I wrote about our relationship because that was really why I done it [sic] … I want them [her friends and family] to know they are reading about our lives. I hope that makes sense to you.

It does. It makes perfect sense, and, even if I were creating of Becky's life a play, a script to be performed, rather than articulating a very real and raw experience in as truthful a way as I can, her illness could not take the lead role. Even in dramatic fiction, where operating theatres transmorph into stage sets and where reality is suspended for art's sake, it is the power of human relationships and the strength of conviction in the face of adversity that must always dictate the underlying plot. That said, this is not a stage set; this is the summer of 2007.

> *Finally the summer was here. Everyone walking round with smiles on their faces because the sun was shining. The sun makes everyone feel better. Well it makes me feel better. A lot goes on in the summer months with birthdays and weddings; it's either meals out getting fatter or nights out getting drunk. Me and Matthew were spending a lot of time together, which was real nice. My parents were really fond of Matthew and his parents were fond of me. It's good when everyone gets on. It's half the battle.*

But, in many ways, for Becky and for Matthew the battle was only just beginning.

Extreme remedies are very appropriate for extreme diseases.

Hippocrates

Vulval Neoplasia

Vulval neoplasia is a term used to define diagnoses both of vulval intraepithelial neoplasia (VIN) and of carcinoma of the vulva, or vulval cancer. The latter is a rare condition but nevertheless accounts for 3–5 per cent of all gynaecological malignancies in the UK. Data collected by Cancer Research UK in 2014–2016 showed that there are approximately 1,300 new vulval cancer cases in the UK every year and the incidence and mortality rates for vulval cancer in the UK are highest in females over 90 years of age. A women's risk of developing cancer depends on many factors, including age, genetics and exposure to risk factors, but the younger a woman is when diagnosed, the better her chances of surviving the cancer for five years or more.

Neoplasia literally means the abnormal proliferation of cells, and in the case of VIN, where abnormal cells are present in a woman's vulva, there is the potential for them to develop into cancer if left untreated. Symptoms of VIN include itching and/or burning sensations in the area, an unpleasant odour and sometimes bleeding from an ulcer or a lump. Standard intervention in such cases usually favours the surgical removal of the affected part by local excision or laser vapourisation (cutting or burning away the affected area), a partial or radical vulvectomy (the removal of half or the whole of the woman's vulva) or, where lymph nodes are involved and depending on the stage of the disease, inguinofemoral lymph node dissection (the complete removal of the lymph nodes all around the affected area). Such intervention is inevitably problematic, most directly because the delicate nature of the woman's anatomy makes even the smallest surgical procedure susceptible to post-operative complications. Moreover, where the rate of recurrence of the disease is up to 50 per cent, the necessary repetition of surgical intervention has inevitable and significant impact on the patient's physical and emotional quality of life. Psychosexual problems are very common.

It Begins

Dr T's sudden appearance at the door of the room brings the outside world into focus and shatters my quiet reverie. She is late, flustered. Only 15 minutes ago she was in theatre finishing up an operation that had turned out to be more complex than expected and now she looks tired, maybe a little anxious. As I get up to greet her, the shards of my thoughts, unformed and fragile as they are, fall around me, even as Dr T seems to gather her own and shrugs off any disquiet that remains about her morning's work. She grins happily on seeing me and we hug, briefly, urgently. Then, after a rushed conversation about what is about to happen, and with a roll of her eyes towards the gathering crowd of women in the waiting area, she leaves as suddenly as she arrived, diving into the organised chaos of her own office. Through the wall I hear the rustling of papers and the sound of the computer coming to life. And so it begins. I close the door, quietly, and wait.

I am in the vulval intraepithelial neoplasia, or VIN, clinic, which occupies a small suite of rooms in the Women's Centre at Llandough Hospital, in Cardiff. Part of the Cardiff and Vale University Health Board, Llandough is the second largest hospital in the city and its mission, as stated on its website, is, perhaps unsurprisingly, all about 'Caring for People, Keeping People Well'. Today, the mission is being accomplished at the Women's Centre as patients at all stages of their treatment for vulval disease come to see their respective consultants. Dr T's list includes those women who have just been diagnosed, as well as those who have come for post-surgical follow-up appointments. Our idea is for her to ask the women, once the consultation is over, whether they would like to talk with me about their experiences of their condition and the treatment measures that they are undergoing, but this is all new territory: nothing is certain and we have no idea whether anybody will agree to be involved. This is the very beginning of the *Drawing Women's Cancer* project. It is early 2012.

But let's go back a bit.

How to cite this book chapter:
Saorsa, J. with Phillips, R. 2019. *Like Any Other Woman: The Lived Experience of Gynaecological Cancer.* Pp. 11–14. Cardiff: Cardiff University Press. DOI: https://doi.org/10.18573/book2.c. License: CC-BY-NC-ND 4.0

I arrive at the clinic early, 20 minutes or so before the afternoon session is due to start, and there are already women sitting in the waiting area. Some are chatting, but overall there is a muted, heavy atmosphere in the room, broken intermittently by the strident ring of the telephone. Dr T is not here, it seems, so I introduce myself to the receptionist at the desk. A middle-aged lady with dark hair that is just beginning to grey, she has a much-practised smile. When she realises I am not a patient, however, her cheeriness wavers a little as she looks anxiously over my shoulder at the increasing number of women coming into the clinic. Nevertheless, she maintains a businesslike air as she lets me know that she's been expecting me and has found a place where I will be able to talk with the patients in private. As she shows me to a small room directly adjacent to the office where Dr T will see her patients, she becomes curious as to what exactly I will be doing. Her questions are polite and she nods and makes murmurs that sound like approval as I stumble through an explanation, but I sense that she is uneasy about accommodating someone who calls herself an artist and, above all, is not medically qualified. (In retrospect, this was to become a common reaction among the medical professionals and hospital staff. An implacable scepticism about the value of what I do is often thinly veiled, and even now, a few years on, although I am gaining ground all the time in terms of increased levels of trust, this is still often accompanied by a wary interest in what the outcome of my work will be.)

Aesthetically bare, and with no windows, the room I am shown into feels a little claustrophobic. The grey carpet is worn and stained in places. It bears a history of people's entrances and exits over the years as they have, in here, sat down to tell their stories and to be told, with breath held for the moment of truth, the results of tests and biopsies. All of their relief, their disappointments, all of their hopes and their fears about their own mortality remain here as quiet whispers and fleeting shadows of meaningful, yet interrupted, lives. These walls, painted with cold and indifferent greyish-blue colour, give little comfort although they harbour so much emotion. Some of the paint is peeling around the doorframe, but it reveals no warmth or respite from the relentless neutrality, just a powdery fragment of dirty white plaster, and even the door itself is painted in the same greyish blue as the walls. It is also a very heavy door, and I discover that it will close by itself, with a bang, unless it is propped open. The short wooden wedge that I find in the corner of the room is presumably there for that very purpose. I notice too the Yale lock, unusual perhaps for an internal door and strangely ominous, but I tell myself that it must be there simply to assure a level of privacy. In the same way, the frosted glass panel at head height is obviously not for looking through. It lets in only a modicum of filtered light, which does little to soften the harsh glare of the fluorescent strip that is softly buzzing on the ceiling.

The room is set up in the familiar consulting room style, but despite the stains on the carpet it doesn't look as if it is used very much. There is nothing here to suggest a regular occupant, and in fact there is nothing to distinguish this grey, impersonal space from any other consulting room in any other part of the hospital, except perhaps for the somewhat random posters about women's health that are tacked onto the wall. Just inside the door and pushed up against the wall there is a desk, ink-stained and scratched like a desk in a school classroom. There are two chairs by it, and the one in front of the desk is large and upholstered in fake black leather. It rocks and swivels and it has a padded headrest. The other chair, at the side of the desk and clearly intended for the patient, is smaller. It is made of plastic and it looks hard and uncomfortable. Opposite the desk, standing heavily against the back wall of the room, are two grey metal filing cabinets, each one supporting a stack of books and what look like medical catalogues on top of it, and on the wall between the desk and these cabinets, where it feels like there should have been a window, there is a sink with a tarnished mirror above. A second 'patient's' chair is positioned awkwardly beside the sink. It looks out of place, obviously there primarily for convenience should someone other than the doctor and the patient be present. The only other thing in the room is a clock above the desk. It is showing the wrong time, but it ticks, loudly. The instinctive yet slightly depressing familiarity of the hierarchical set-up in this drab and uninspiring room makes me want to rebel and rearrange the furniture. I feel the need, it is visceral, but I curb the impulse and try to convince myself, not without a twinge of guilt, that my choice to sit in the larger chair is purely based on comfort.

The waiting area is filling up with patients now. Two other consultants are on duty along with Dr T, and there are also appointments scheduled with specialist nurses. I can hear a murmuring of voices and a scraping of chairs resonating from the next room as Dr T greets her first patient. I can only wait.

Dr T is naturally optimistic. During the many meetings we had to organise this visit she was always confident that her patients would be willing to get involved. I am less so, but hopeful, and now, waiting here alone in this drab room, I wonder how things will turn out. The murmuring continues. What news is the patient being given? Has the surgery gone well? If it was VIN, has the progression of the disease been halted? If it was cancer, has the tumour been removed? What next? Has pre-cancer developed into cancer itself? Might it even already have been cancer?

As the moments go by, every second announced by the loud ticking of the clock, I begin to feel self-conscious, out of place, heavy-limbed in the chair, almost as if I am myself the patient. I check, just as I have done several times that day, that the voice recorder is set up correctly and that the batteries are good. I fidget with my notebook and scribble to make sure the pen works, even though I don't really anticipate making any notes during the conversation because, somehow, it doesn't feel either right or respectful to do so. I pick up a stray paperclip that is lying on the desk and start to play with it, twisting and distorting it out of shape. It's a habit of mine, a sort of idle manipulation of a pliant material that fulfils a need in me to have something to occupy my hands.

Perhaps such 'fiddling' is a way of relocating my fundamental artist-self in an environment that is, essentially, alien. The sculptural form of the contorted paperclip, a complex arrangement of tiny steel triangles, now sits before me on the desk and its presence is strangely comforting. As I look at it I begin to feel more at ease.

It feels like an age, but actually I have to wait for only 10 minutes before the murmuring stops in the office next door. Then, just as suddenly as she had appeared earlier, Dr T bursts excitedly into the room and introduces me to the first patient who has agreed to see me. Her name is Rebecca.

I was not looking for my dreams to interpret my life,
but rather for my life to interpret my dreams.

Susan Sontag

Meeting Becky

It's a cold November night in 2012 and I'm having difficulty sleeping. I'm thinking to myself I would like to share my story of what's gone on in my life over the past couple of years, some real good and some not so good. My name is Rebecca Phillips, some know me as Becky, and I'm twenty-seven years old. I met my husband, Matthew, over nine years ago and for the first couple of years things wasn't that serious between us because you know what boys are like, they want to be with their friends and they want a girlfriend. The friends always win... but that's another story.

From 2006 things got real serious between us because unfortunately a dreadful thing happened. Matthew's best friend, Craig, was killed doing his everyday job that he loved. When that happened I think it made Matthew realise life was too short. He missed Craig so much and I was always there for him when he wanted to talk. Not long before Craig died he said something to Matthew that will always stay with him, he said that Matthew would be with me for the rest of his life. This is where our journey, Matthew's and mine begins. Matthew became a different person after everything that had happened. I was his rock and he was my rock. I couldn't have asked for a better husband.

Rebecca, or Becky as I am to discover she prefers to be called, enters the room with a confident air. She is followed by her mother, 'Mam', who is less self-assured and remains, hovering, in the doorway. Mam always comes to support Becky during the hospital appointments. Her love and protectiveness for her daughter is evident in the tender way she looks at her, but the look is also tempered by the worry and stress that Becky's illness has caused over the months. I am to find out later, while talking with Becky, that there has been a long history of serious illness, mainly cancer, in the extended family and this has inevitably taken its toll. There is little wonder then that Mam appears so anxious about anything new.

How to cite this book chapter:
Saorsa, J. with Phillips, R. 2019. *Like Any Other Woman: The Lived Experience of Gynaecological Cancer.* Pp. 17–23. Cardiff: Cardiff University Press. DOI: https://doi.org/10.18573/book2.d. License: CC-BY-NC-ND 4.0

After polite introductions and we have all shaken hands, Dr T takes her leave. One of the nurses is calling the second patient on her list and she has many to attend to this session. I hear her usher the woman into her office and shut the door as I quickly pull up the spare chair and invite Becky and Mam to sit down.

Becky is smiling broadly but Mam, still by the door, hesitates. She seems reluctant to commit to this new development, but, perhaps unwilling to voice her concerns because it is clear that Becky is entirely happy to be involved, she makes no comment. There is a momentary awkwardness as something passes between them, unsaid, and then, with a final anxious glance towards her daughter and a polite nod towards me, Mam discreetly leaves the room.

Becky seems expectant, even excited, not just willing but positively eager to talk to me. She is very pretty and looks remarkably healthy given what she has been through. Her youthful features and almost playful demeanour belie even her 26 years and are, I've since learnt, the hallmarks of her engaging personality. Indeed, the room, poorly lit as it is, seems suddenly brighter with her presence. Neither tall nor noticeably short, she is of average height and build, and despite the physical and emotional difficulties that her condition has necessarily imposed, she still exudes the confidence and the optimism of youth. She has clearly spent a lot of time on her appearance. Her expressive face carries a light layer of make-up, barely discernible, but her lips are defined by a glossy slash of deep crimson lipstick, so rich it seems as if it is the only real colour in the otherwise drab room. Her hair is short and very, boldly, blonde. The cut suits her. Straight at the nape of her neck and over her ears, with a thick fringe that threatens to fall heavily over her forehead but is swept extravagantly to the side and held there, in suspended animation, by some imperceptible force. She is wearing a short black jacket over a light-coloured dress and a scarf that looks like natural linen is loosely draped around her neck. Her surprisingly small feet are elegantly clothed in a pair of short, black leather boots.

As Becky sits down, carefully but without hesitation, I notice the deliberate way she moves, slower than would seem normal and with an obvious consciousness of her body. Her original operation, which involved the complete removal of her vulva followed by a reconstruction using flesh from her buttocks, was carried out two years ago, in 2010, but just three weeks ago she underwent an operation to reverse the colostomy that the original operation had necessitated. I wait until she is settled before sitting down myself, and she chooses the chair at the side of the desk, leaving me to return to the larger chair in front of it. In doing so she quite naturally, instinctively perhaps, sets up the accustomed doctor–patient scenario, and the situation does make me feel slightly awkward until I inwardly chide myself for making too much of its significance. After all, I had been sitting in the larger chair in the first place, and, more importantly, Becky doesn't appear to be in the least bit uncomfortable with the arrangement. She is keen to talk to me and quickly lets me know how disappointed she is that the doctor she had actually come to see was not there and so she has to rearrange her appointment. She says, a little shyly, 'I was supposed to see Dr D today...' She pauses, and when she begins again her voice is low. She is staring at the floor as if she is embarrassed. 'I need to see him because my bum has got... well, a little fatty at the bottom.'

I wonder, aloud, why she had not been informed of Dr D's absence before she came for the appointment, especially as it was to arrange a surgical procedure, one which, as I am to find out later, would be only one of many that she has had over the last couple of years. Becky only continues to stare at her boots. This is the first time in our short acquaintance that I have seen any sign of emotional pain. Finally she looks up and says that, as Dr T had been able to give her only a few minutes in-between other ladies who were on her own list, she is glad to talk with me since, at the very least, it means that her long journey to the hospital has not been for nothing. I assure her that I am delighted she has agreed to speak with me and I turn on the voice recorder.

'I'm Rebecca ... I'm 26 years old. I got diagnosed with vulval cancer in 2010.'

She has a characteristically lilting tone of voice that resonates with her upbringing in the Rhondda Valley, here in South Wales. Her strong and unmistakable accent emphasises and lengthens the vowel sounds, as certain consonants get lost in the flow. She begins her story by telling me that she was diagnosed with vulval cancer two years ago when she was just 24, and as she continues to speak, in a surprisingly matter-of-fact way about something that must have been devastating at the time, I begin to understand how much this bright young woman has had to contend with over the last couple of years. Her diagnosis was even more devastating perhaps because, while there can never be a right time for such an assault on a person's sense of self as a cancer diagnosis, in Becky's case it was especially cruel as it came only four months before her planned wedding.

During the course of the *Drawing Women's Cancer* project, and since meeting Becky, I have attended many operations and all are burnt into my memory due to the nature of what I have witnessed, and to the generosity and trust afforded me by the women patients who allowed me to be there. Looking back now in retrospect it was clear that, while talking to me in the small, bare room at the women's clinic, even two years after her own procedure, the experience for Becky was still very powerfully fresh in her mind. The original surgery was effective in ridding her of cancer, but the physical and emotional effects of such a major operation, and the problems she is still experiencing due to its consequences, have dramatically changed the way that she lives her young life.

> Hairdresser, I was. I worked really hard. I'm going back to it though. I thought I'd be back in a week after the operation, but I never did go. I went from a really, really busy life to nothing... nothing at all.

I begin to feel profoundly sad as Becky relives her disappointment at not being able to continue at the hair salon. It is a shared sadness, of course, and I feel a profound empathy as she tells me how she had loved her job and how it had brought her out of herself, given her a confidence she had never had as a child. But her busy life, close to perfect in its fulfilment of everything she had ever felt she wanted, has, with the illness, come to a 'standstill', and in the time that she now has too much of, thinking about how her whole world has changed, she worries about what she sees as the waste of her youth, the loss of the confidence that she had battled so hard to gain and the anguish that she fears her angry outbursts, albeit brief and infrequent, might now be causing her husband and her family.

> I get annoyed with myself. I do. I have off days and I get annoyed with myself when I want to do something and I can't. Then someone will say, 'Let me do it for you', and I'll snap their heads off then. No, I'm not very nice to them and sometimes I'll shout, 'Just leave me alone!' I know they only want to help – but you don't like to depend on somebody all the time.

She tells me of her embarrassment about the weight she has put on since the original operation. 'I look like a different person in the mirror. I don't feel like a different person but I put on two stone in weight and because of my operation I had a real big bum as well, it was really swollen. The doctor said about 18 months, but 18 months is a long time. Like, I've tried so hard to lose weight. I'm doing a little bit of walking. I'm not a lazy person anyway. When I came out of hospital I went mad on food, I was always hungry but not big meals; I just fancied junk food basically.' Becky paints a picture for me in words of a young woman sitting alone in her bedroom crying softly to herself because she cannot squeeze into the jeans that she wore before the operation. And even though the picture does no justice to the young woman who now sits before me, with her shiny red lips and her elegant outfit, it is clear nevertheless that for her, as for anybody who feels deeply, the profound disappointment and carefully guarded sense of unfairness that characterises her experience can sometimes dissolve into despair. A shadow moved over her sun, just as a tumour casts its shadow over the MRI.

Suddenly Becky rallies herself, just the way I suspect she has been doing repeatedly over the last couple of years. She shifts impatiently in her chair as if physically shaking off the spectre of the girl on the bed. 'I will never give up,' she says. 'I'm too young for that.' I believe her. With my gentle prompting she begins to tell me, from the beginning, what she's been through, and I sense that we are together building a mutual trust.

Becky says that when she was given the original diagnosis of vulval cancer she was less worried for herself than for Matthew, her future husband, and for her family, and, in any case, 'I was numb. In a daze.' It is clear that at the time, she wanted to disassociate herself from the worry and the fear of what might be in store and tried to do so by focusing on recognising it only in those close to her. I know instinctively however that it would be a very disrespectful mistake to think that this was a fully conscious level of transference, or even just a way of avoiding facing up to the inevitable. Becky's sense of family love and loyalty is so strong and pervasive in everything she is telling me that I begin to understand how this has played a central role in helping her manage to get through the trials of recent years as the assaults on both her physical and emotional being have been increasingly harsh and seemingly unrelenting.

As she tells me about the initial diagnosis of vulval cancer and the preparations for her operation, Becky maintains her confident air. It is almost as if she is talking about something far more innocuous than the actual traumatic event she is describing. I notice however that her smile does waver a little as she tells me that the only thing that she could not push away from her mind at the time was the dread of having to have a colostomy bag after the surgery. Indeed, the horror of it still plays tricks with her sense of equilibrium, but, as she has done for nearly all of the experiences she has gone through, at the time she put all her faith in the doctors. Even on the morning of the procedure the only question she had was about the chances of her waking up with a colostomy bag. The answer came like a physical blow: 90 per cent.

She underwent a full, radical vulvectomy followed by plastic surgery for reconstruction. Maybe due to not asking many questions, maybe due to not understanding all of the information she was given, or maybe because of sheer, innocent, blind trust, she went into the operation not fully realising the extent of what was going to be done. Her innocence made for a harsh awakening. 'I had to have a lot of plastic surgery done. Quite a lot of skin was removed from my bum cheeks – both sides. But they kept...' here she pauses. It is hard for her to keep the veneer of confidence intact. 'The top half is my own. Because of my age, I think, because I haven't got children yet.' As she pauses again, just for a moment, she is clearly thinking again of what she discovered that fateful afternoon and a cloud passes over her pretty face. Then she whispers, 'My whole life turned upside down.'

There follows a silence between us that seems to settle over us like a blanket, but it is not uncomfortable. Even though I hardly know this young woman, and even though she is telling me things that must be as difficult for her to talk about as they are for me to listen to, she has created an atmosphere of unadulterated honesty, genuineness and trust. And the small room, at first devoid of much humanity, now feels warmer and richer for it. Suddenly, unexpectedly, Becky smiles and the blanket lifts. No, it's not a smile; it's a cheeky grin! She says, 'I'm still able to have sex.' I say, 'Well that's good to hear,' and we laugh. We laugh as two women might do who understand that they share something more than is within the words said. Becky continues, upbeat now and very much in touch with her story. She tells me that she was in hospital for 10 days after her operation and, as it was still difficult for her to walk when she came home, she needed a wheelchair to get around. Nevertheless, two weeks after leaving hospital, and with her mother to help her, she went shopping. 'I did my hair, put on make-up. I always want to look nice. I felt better.'

But it couldn't always be OK. Just as fast as it had brightened, Becky's mood darkens again and she frowns, staring at the floor as if there is a gaping hole at her feet. The harsh light in the room seems to dim, just a little, and it feels almost like she is confessing some aberration as she says,

> I did feel low sometimes and I went to counselling, which helped. I was angry more than anything. I felt all my womanhood had been taken from me. It didn't affect my relationship with Matthew; if anything he is very, very understanding. A lot of men would have run a mile, considering we were so young as well, and we didn't have a very good start in life. But things are much, much better now.

She is as insistent that her counselling sessions helped her through a bad time as she is clear in her wish to recommend counselling in general for anyone in her situation. Meanwhile I am trying hard to only listen and not to be drawn into any kind of therapeutic engagement myself, even though my instincts, and my own professional training in the field, are pushing me towards it. I remind myself that it would be totally inappropriate, but I can't help wondering where the difference really lies. How much can simply talking about human experience with an empathetic listener help a person? How much dissimilarity is there between what is agreed to be counselling, a therapeutic relationship, and a conversation between equals?

Of course, I know the answers to these questions full well. In an active counselling situation I would listen, sometimes guide and sometimes challenge in order to encourage the 'client' to explore alternative ways of thinking about and understanding situations, experiences and feelings, but here, now, in this small, bare room, my intention is to simply listen, and support if necessary. In both situations my primary aim, beyond everything else, is to give the person in front of me (in this case, Becky) the security and the latitude to tell their story in the way that they see it. But such stories are always profound, and, while I am more than willing to allow Becky all the space she needs to tell hers, I am acutely aware that what is really in question here is the level of emotional security. In a professional counselling relationship, where the promise of continuance is tacit, wounds can be opened and feelings explored within the safety of a relationship that is built upon over time. In Becky's case, however, I must be careful to contain the emotion as much as I can within the timeframe of this one meeting. I am unable to promise any return visit. I begin to understand at this moment, more than I ever have during all of the preparation for the project, that this disjunction between what I want to do as a counsellor and what I can do as a person is something I will wrestle with throughout.

Becky is looking forward to trying for a baby, to starting a family of her own. She has been told that there is no reason why she could not get pregnant, but she doesn't want to rush into anything because, as she says, since she's been married it has been 'nothing but hospitals and illness'. But on the other hand, 'I don't want to leave it too long as you don't know what's around the corner'. Then I ask, bluntly, 'Do you trust your body?' Becky hesitates, a little bemused perhaps by the question, or by my directness. She draws herself up and says, 'I do. Yes. And I check myself all the time'. There is another pause and then an even more confident response. 'I trust Dr T. All my trust is in her'.

Mam, who has been waiting in the seating area outside, gets up quickly as Becky and I leave the room. Her anxious look is still there as she automatically reaches out, protectively, toward her daughter. We talk briefly about the project and I reassure them both that Becky has been wonderfully helpful in what we are trying to do. Becky is smiling as I thank her and tell her that I hope we can talk again. They need to go. We've been talking for a long time and the traffic will be building up on the roads out of the city. As they leave through the sliding doors at the entrance to the clinic I have a distinct feeling that something has begun.

But there are two more women who have been patiently waiting to talk with me. I take a deep breath, smile, and approach the first. 'Hello there, is it Jo?'

It's more important to know what sort of person has a disease than to know what sort of disease a person has.

Hippocrates

SUTURE 1: Jo. VIN and AIN

Jo quickly gets up from the chair where she has been sitting, waiting. Short in stature, she is of stocky build and her brown hair is neatly cut into a bob that ends abruptly at her jawline. She looks very young, even for her 28 years, and healthy too; her skin is clear and glowing and there seems only a trace of make-up on her face, if any at all. She returns my smile, but there is still a certain tension in her expression, a strange mixture of hesitancy and determination that sharply defines her otherwise gentle features. I greet her warmly with a handshake and usher her into the small room. She seems nervous, naturally perhaps, but there is a kindness, a compassion in her eyes that assures me that I am in the company of an intelligent and mature young woman, indeed a fellow 'old soul'.

Jo's features soften and she seems to relax once there is a door between her and the open space of the waiting room, and she sits down, carefully placing her bag on the floor by her feet. She is dressed well, stylish but not overtly so, and she has a grace about her movements. But there is something more, something that I can sense but cannot quite bring to consciousness, something about Jo that feels fundamental but which isn't yet in the room. As I sit down opposite her I feel strangely sad.

Trying to shake off premonition, I begin by briefly explaining what we will be doing and about the project. I know that Dr T has already done this but I'm hoping it will break the ice a little. It seems to work. Jo nods in acknowledgement of all I am saying and assures me that she wants to be involved, with the familiar phrase that nearly all of the ladies I have worked with throughout the project seem to habitually use: 'If it helps'. Even so, I notice that she is still eyeing the voice recorder with some suspicion as she begins to tell her story.

> I'm 28 now. I was about 11 when I noticed I was bleeding around my back passage. I didn't think anything of it except that perhaps it was just

normal. But when I was 18 and sexually active, well I can only describe it as this overwhelming burning inside. It put me off, I didn't want to do it because it hurt so bad and because of that I went to the doctor, and then I went through all sorts.'

Jo takes a breath, there is a long pause, and in the silence she seems to retreat into the part of her that I sensed she left outside the door. It is a struggle not to say something, not to try to compensate for the sense of loss that has pervaded the room, but I know that anything I might say just at this moment would seem inane, superfluous, so I remain quiet and simply wait. Jo visibly gathers herself and shifts her position in the chair so that she is directly facing me across the small space between us, which, with that action, has suddenly become even smaller. 'It was quite frustrating really. I was treated for all sorts because they didn't really know what I was talking about. Eventually, it was three years later, I went to see the doctor and she said that she could see some kind of skin complaint all around front and back.'

Jo's diagnosis took a long time coming. Even after the confirmation by her GP of 'some kind of skin complaint', she tells me that it took two further years of treatment before a dermatologist in a hospital in England, but not far from Cardiff, finally took a biopsy and determined the extent of her problems. Jo's account of her experiences feels quite detached, as if she is reporting what happened to someone else, and, other than a reluctance to make full eye contact with me, her manner doesn't allow any outward indication of emotion as she tells me that it was in December 2009, years after her first symptoms began, that she received news that she had a serious pre-cancerous condition called VIN. Indeed, perhaps sensing my thoughts, she goes on to qualify this. 'Actually it was massive relief, because there was one stage when I thought I was going mad – I can't think of another way to put it – a freak of nature, because nobody seemed to know what I was talking about.'

As I listen to Jo I am trying to conceive of the anguish that the feeling she describes of being misunderstood, even disbelieved, must have engendered. It is difficult, especially so because, as she is telling me in such a matter-of-fact way, the emotional content of her account seems to be more a problem for me than for her. Of course it can't be, and I know that I need to simply focus on what she is saying. I have to try hard to take this encounter on Jo's terms.

The afternoon is wearing on and, despite the buzzing tube on the ceiling, the light is fading in the room. There is a slight pause and then, suddenly, Jo says something that I know I will remember for a long time, not because of anything necessarily profound in the words themselves but rather because of the sudden emphasis she places on them, because of the way she finally looks directly at me, because of the fire that burns briefly in her eyes as she recalls the moment she could tell herself with total clarity that she was not a freak of nature. 'I didn't care that I had abnormal cells that might turn into cancer. I had an answer! I had an answer!'

Now, seemingly into her stride, Jo becomes more animated as she tells me about how, once the diagnosis was confirmed, a gynaecologist who specialised in skin conditions arranged for her to have what was to be her first operation to remove the affected skin from her vulva. Even then, because there were logistical 'complications' as to where she would be able to have the operation carried out, it was another year before she actually went into surgery. As I listen I am inwardly questioning how such a delay could even be acceptable in a health system such as ours, let alone be tolerated with as much patience and grace as Jo obviously had. Given that she was a young woman, recently married, and had been suffering for years with this condition under the very noses of those who were supposed to be qualified to help her, the very least they could have offered should surely have been a speedy resolution once the diagnosis was confirmed. But Jo is still talking, fluently now, giving words to thoughts and memories, and she seems almost excited about telling her story. I wonder whether this is the first time she has really been given the opportunity to do so before I chide myself for allowing my own thoughts to again override my ability to actually listen. It is her words that are important here, not mine, and so I nod, smile, and make what I hope are reassuring and encouraging noises as she continues, and I listen harder.

> He took some of the skin away from the one section and joined the rest together. He said it was a fairly simple operation. It did mean that I was bed bound for a couple of weeks because, well, the only way I can describe it is like when a woman tears badly during childbirth. The worst part was going to the loo. It was like razor blades. And it didn't just affect the front. He had to take some away from the back as well. I had to take painkillers and wait 20 minutes for them to work before going to the loo. The pain was horrendous.

Here, despite my steadfast resolve to focus entirely on what Jo is saying, my own internal questioning starts, annoyingly, again. Her description of complications in childbirth feels odd, as I know she has no children as yet, but it also pulls aspects of my own history out from the shadows within which old pain often sleeps, awaiting a telling. I do know exactly how and what she must be imagining actually feels. But this is not about me! It is about Jo! And I now feel guilty as she wavers just a little and hesitates after what has been an almost continuous flow of words. Did she notice my absence, if only for a moment? She stammers a little. 'I-I'm just trying to remember the sequence of events.' Anxiety now becomes a visible emotion etched over her youthful features as she tells me that six months after her first operation she was still suffering with pain and soreness, away from the vulval area now and more around her anus. A second operation confirmed that not only did she have VIN (vulval intraepithelial neoplasia) but AIN (anal epithelial neoplasia) as well.

That part of her left outside the room has definitely made its entrance now and it wants to tell its story in the angry and emotional terms that, even though Jo wouldn't like to admit it, must, ultimately, give credence to her autonomous self. For too many years, indeed since childhood, she has felt isolated and alone in suffering a condition that she felt nobody understood, even to the point that she feared she might be losing her mind. And now she is telling me that even when she was diagnosed she still felt alone and abandoned by the system.

> I was angry. At the Bath hospital where they diagnosed it [AIN], they knew what it was but they didn't really know anything about it so they couldn't treat me. I'd say to myself, 'God, these are medical professionals who are supposed to know about everything and they can't help me!' I remember him [her consultant] telling me he could confirm AIN but then saying basically that he couldn't do anything more for me. I remember walking out of the consultation and nearly bursting into tears … I thought, isn't anybody going to do anything about this then?

Painfully for us both I drew out the word that was struggling to breathe from the emotion that pervaded the room. I read it aloud as if it were written on her forehead.

'Abandoned?'

'Yes!'

Her answer is clear, if still ambiguous in nature. She is assertive on the surface but there is a fragile bridge between courage and defiance over a deep sea of vulnerability. Looking directly at me again, she says, 'I'm actually pregnant now. We don't know yet which way it's going to go. I've had a scan, its underdeveloped, but for someone with VIN I never thought I'd be able to… because it is so painful… so if this fails I can carry on again.'

Something seems to change between us just at that moment, just as Jo tells me of her pregnancy. I feel as if I've been let into a secret, and I warm to the level of trust that she must surely have in me to talk about this. I remind myself inwardly of the need to simply let her say whatever she needs to say without interrupting too much, the need for me to simply be there, and listen. There is, however, a short pause and Jo looks down again, at her shoes. She is perhaps gathering her thoughts, and I am hoping that she appreciates my silence as an indication of my understanding of her need to do so. In the silence between us it seems as if the clock in the room has suddenly started to tick even more loudly while the sounds from the busy clinic on the other side of the door disappear into what feels like a temporal vacuum. I wonder anxiously whether the same vacuum will suck both of us in too, but finally, and suddenly, Jo says something that surprises me in its quiet and conciliatory nature. This does not feel like the painful truth of a moment ago; it feels more like an attempt to shore up the emotion that she is clearly feeling. 'Time is a great healer. It's a lot better now and I've got hardly any symptoms. I come here now every six months to have it checked because there's still some… they can't get rid of all of it... just to make sure that it doesn't turn cancerous.' Jo looks at me. Her expression has softened. Is it a hopeful look? Am I wrong in sensing that she is looking imploringly? Does she want reassurance, confirmation that the future is bright, cancer free? Then she continues, 'So, there is light at the end of the tunnel and at times now I wouldn't even know that I've got abnormal skin.'

The clichés continue to fall, crashing against all sense of vulnerability and shoring up any cracks that might let loose the emotion I witnessed earlier. The trite themes drip almost apologetically from her lips, which themselves describe an uncomfortable and unconvincing smile. I feel a rise of panic because it seems as if I am losing her, just as I thought she trusted me. Was it something that I had said? Something I didn't say? I feign interest and conformity under involuntarily raised eyebrows, but, even as I silently castigate myself for being less than honest, something unspoken passes between us and Jo's manner changes. She shifts again in her chair and seems to come to a decision. I know that I have to earn trust; it is a gift more easily received than given, but my fear that I may have lost Jo's trust now vanishes as she says,

> As far as the VIN goes it wasn't a major case, but it was enough to make somebody almost lose the will to live sometimes. I just didn't know what it was and the amount of times I was with my husband and we tried and I was in tears because I just couldn't go through with it, that was just awful.

I am always humbled by the amount of trust granted me by all the women I work with, and in this moment I feel Jo has assuredly gifted me with hers. She says,

> It's very difficult when people ask what my operations were for. I just say, 'Well...' At first it was difficult because I was only about 19. It was very undignified. Back then I'd just started a job as a childcare officer for the local authority. It didn't have any bearing on my work life until the operations. I didn't want to share with too many people, especially as we've got one male and if he asks, well you don't feel like you can explain it because he will never understand what you're talking about. I was silly. I went to the hospital appointment thinking I could handle it all, the same as all those times I went to the doctors and they said, 'Well we don't know what it is. Try these creams.' And after all this, someone telling me that there's nothing more they can do for me. I couldn't speak about it to anyone. There was only my husband and there was a time when I couldn't have a physical relationship with him for nearly a year. And he was really understanding. I'm lucky. It was awful. I couldn't even go to my friends and expect them to understand it because they'd never heard of VIN. But it's not until I retell the story, like now, that I realise what a journey it's been.

There is a pause while both of us reflect on everything she's just said, and then I ask a single question. 'Has it changed you?' Jo is ready for it. The determined look in her eye has returned. The light has come back.

It's made me stronger. How can I explain it? Well, I coped with the two operations very well. I was just in and out. I was up and eating a sandwich just half an hour after! I just kept going I thought this isn't going to beat me so it has made me stronger. I cope with things much better now because of it and I don't give up – I'm determined. What gave me the strength was knowing deep down that I wasn't going mad. I knew that there was something wrong and I kept on to people until they did something. The relief when I came around the corner here and there was a sign that said VIN clinic! My mum actually took a picture of it. At times in the past I would see my body as the enemy. But now, because the symptoms have subsided quite a bit, life is all right at the moment. I still get the feeling sometimes that people don't understand but they never will because even though its more well known now, VIN, only vulval… I can't say it – it's too scientific – so that doesn't help at all! There needs to be a simplified name. You think, Oh! I've got this thing and I can't pronounce it! My attitude changed after I came here. Things have got better, physically. My husband has understood. He's always been very positive. He's pushed me along really. I don't think he's going to be very happy when I tell him the baby is underdeveloped. We'll cross that bridge when we come to it. I'll either lose it or I won't. I'll try again. Keep at it. That's a thing I would say to anybody who is going through this… don't give up. You know your body.

The Senedd Exhibition, 2012: Speaking the Unspeakable

You're having an exhibition on vulval cancer? What, open to the public? With drawings? Blimey!
Member of public on hearing about the exhibition

For want of awareness – For want of openness – For want of a shared experience

Speaking the Unspeakable, the first exhibition for the *Drawing Women's Cancer* project, took place at the Senedd, the Welsh Assembly building that majestically overlooks Cardiff Bay, in the evening of 22 November 2012. It was a Thursday.

This was never intended to be a conventional exhibition, never just about putting pictures on a wall, about simply looking. This exhibition was about encouraging everyone there to talk about vulval cancer, a condition that had somehow been sidestepped by the publicity machines that had recently gone into overdrive around the death in 2009 of a celebrity, Jade Goody, who had suffered a related illness, cervical cancer. Even now at the time of writing, in 2018, public awareness of cervical cancer is considerable while the suffering caused by vulval cancer remains, if not unrecognised, still far less acknowledged. In fact, although vulval cancer is a comparatively rare form of gynaecological disease, and is often considered by those who do acknowledge it as primarily one that affects older women, it actually accounts for 3–5 per cent of genealogical malignancies in the UK and affects women at both ends of the age spectrum. Becky and Jo, diagnosed in their twenties with vulval cancer and VIN, respectively, are living proof of this hard fact.

Cardiff huddled under a deluge on that winter evening. Howling winds and torrential rain drowned out the noise of the city and created an almost theatrical

How to cite this book chapter:
Saorsa, J. with Phillips, R. 2019. *Like Any Other Woman: The Lived Experience of Gynaecological Cancer.* Pp. 31–33. Cardiff: Cardiff University Press.
DOI: https://doi.org/10.18573/book2.f. License: CC-BY-NC-ND 4.0

atmosphere. It felt as if the downpour would never let up as we peered through the darkened, plate glass windows of the Senedd onto a shallow lake that was rapidly forming in the low amphitheatre of the Bay. I was too anxious, too convinced that the evening would be a literal washout. I was suffering the usual vague nausea that I experience on every opening night when my work is on the wall and I am metaphorically laid bare, but this time it felt more acute as the exhibition was less about me than about the women I really didn't want to let down.

Everything was prepared. The work hung lightly on the walls and the guest book lay open on the desk with pens provided. There was even a box and notecards so that people could write comments that they might prefer to remain private. 'Nibbles' were laid out temptingly on the table and glasses stood in regimental rows, ready to be filled either with wine or any of three different kinds of fruit juice. We needed only the guests. And then they came! With wet coats, wet hair and with stories of huge tailbacks on the M4 that left traffic at a total standstill in the city centre, they came to fill the hall with their chatter and with their supportive and genuine interest in the project. My relief was tangible. People came that night in far greater numbers than we had ever expected. Politicians, medics, patients and their families, members of the public. Becky drove down with her family, despite the weather, from her small hometown in the Valleys. She was excited, happy. She posed for pictures in front of the artwork and she talked, so much and to so many people. She told them all, including the politicians and the policy makers, about the experiences she had gone through since diagnosis. Most seemed to listen, some just politely but many with genuine interest, and Becky was in her element. The people came to see, to understand, because before they came vulval disease was invisible, inaudible and 'without a voice'. That night, the exhibition encouraged everybody to begin 'speaking the unspeakable'.

Dr T spoke about the nature of vulval disease.

'No one can see it. No one can hear it. No one talks about it.'

Our two guest speakers spoke eloquently. The Minister for Health and Social Services, Lesley Griffiths, said,

> Cancer is increasingly becoming a chronic condition people can live with, however, that does not lessen the impact it has on the lives of people who fight and survive it. This exhibition is not only unique; it is emotive and thought-provoking. It gives an insight to the torrent of emotions a woman might experience when she has been diagnosed with a gynaecological cancer in a visual and interactive way.

And the Chief Nursing Officer, Dr Jean White, said,

> Clinically, more and more people survive cancer. However, the emotional trauma a woman may go through when faced with the prospect of

physical changes to her body cannot be underestimated. The exhibition is a physical expression of the psychological effects cancer can have, and I think it will resonate with many people. It is important that services respond holistically to people's needs and preferences.

That night we broke the silence.

As to diseases, make a habit of two things—to help, or at least to do no harm.

Hippocrates

Becky. Return Visit: Part 1

Just short of a year after the exhibition at the Senedd, in September 2013, I visited Becky again. She seemed delighted when I contacted her to ask if she would be able to meet with me and immediately invited me to visit her at home. She was still unwell and, as she lives some distance from the city, such an arrangement was more convenient from her point of view, but there was something else about the invitation, something that I was very conscious of, and grateful for. It was surely a declaration of trust that she would allow me into her home, into her life, in this very personal way.

On the day of my visit it is raining, hard, and it reminds me of the night of the exhibition launch in the Senedd. The 'Valleys' are some distance from Cardiff, and as I drive away from the urban clutches of the city and enter a quieter, more rural landscape the Welsh countryside begins to surround me, brooding and unfamiliar. The damp stillness in the air is broken only by the falling rain and the frantic motion of the windscreen wipers jerking backwards and forwards in a Sisyphean effort to pull back the curtain of rain that constantly closes on the glass. The sound of them is hypnotic and makes me drowsy. I feel a great sense of relief as I finally arrive at the fringes of Becky's hometown. The main street, a primary artery, is lined with grey brick houses and empty shop fronts. Everything looks run down and, deserted as it is in this foul weather, the sense of the town's lifeblood having been drained away is strong. Historically, this town was just a rural hamlet until the second half of the 19th century, when the market for coal and steel spread work and wealth across the whole of the South Wales region. But things have changed and now the industrial villages, the communities that fostered pride and self-reliance in an unforgiving landscape, have become shadows of their former selves.

The rain begins to abate as I turn off the main street and drive up a short incline into the modern estate that stands above the town. This is where Becky lives. There is more open space here, more light, even though the sky remains a cold, stubborn grey and seems to hover low and malignant over the wet

How to cite this book chapter:
Saorsa, J. with Phillips, R. 2019. *Like Any Other Woman: The Lived Experience of Gynaecological Cancer*. Pp. 35–39. Cardiff: Cardiff University Press.
DOI: https://doi.org/10.18573/book2.g. License: CC-BY-NC-ND 4.0

pavements. The houses look very alike, mostly semi-detached, although there are some larger, detached properties, and they are set back behind clean pavements and neatly maintained grass verges that border streets with names ending in 'Close' or 'Walk'. Most of the houses are fronted by neat and thoughtfully planted squares of garden. Hardy shrubs and perennials surround regularly trimmed lawns that are precisely edged and sometimes sport a centrepiece, a red Japanese acer, a blue conifer, all thriving in the damp climate. There are not many cars in the driveways and some of the houses have curtains drawn. Unemployment is high and harsh in the Valleys, but I suspect that here, just now, at three in the afternoon, many of these houses are empty, save for the young and the old. Commuting to work has become necessary and commonplace in this decimated section of post-industrial society, but for those whose lives were never so dictated by coal and steel, as were the lives of their forebears, the two major conurbations of Cardiff and Swansea are not so far away.

The numbers on the houses are difficult to see through the car window so I park at the top of Becky's street and start to walk back, peering at the doors to orientate myself as the rain begins again in earnest and a cold wind picks up. It blows the stinging shards of rain straight into my face, and, semi-blind, I walk straight past the house I'm looking for because my view of where I'm going is reduced to a watery vista of a street full of houses that all look the same. Eventually I turn around, and with the wind now blowing me back up the street I retrace my confused steps and finally arrive at Becky's door. It is already open and Becky is standing just inside, waiting for me, smiling the same broad smile that she gifted me the very first time we met in the clinic at the hospital. 'I seen you go by!' she says and ushers me inside. I feel a little foolish as water drips from my wet clothes onto her hall carpet.

In the living room a gas fire is softly glowing and warm. Becky offers me a towel. Mam is there with her, and her little dog, a dachshund, is barking valiantly even as he is picked up and put firmly into the kitchen. From there, and behind a closed door, 'Charlie' still makes his presence felt, and although I gently protest that I don't mind dogs at all Mam is adamant that he is 'noisy'. (On reading Becky's writing soon after this meeting I discover how important this vocal little dog, Charlie, has been for both her and for her family.)

> I have had dogs all my life and one dog that I have always loved since I was a little girl was a sausage dog. Matthew was warming to the idea. I asked my parents what they thought and they said, 'Why not?' From that night I was looking on the Internet and I came across dachshunds for sale in Carmarthen. I rang the number but when I spoke to the lady who was breeding them I really didn't like her attitude. It sounded a bit, well... not right. I thought, 'This is a puppy farm' so it put me straight off. I'm a massive dog lover and I certainly do not agree with puppy farms. I couldn't find anything else but I kept on looking and when we went up my parents house early one Sunday morning I was looking through the paper to see if

there were any dogs for sale and I found a tiny square advert for miniature dachshunds. There were no photos so I had a little read and the person only lived twenty minutes away. I rang the number and had a chat with the lady who told me she had only one dog left and he was a boy. We went to have a look at him. I was so excited when we got there and we seen him. We fell in love! He was so little and cute. There and then we decided we wanted him but we didn't have anything in the house so I had to go and get everything ready for him. We decided to call him Charlie. That day was a really happy day for us. Charlie was our baby, and he still is. He is spoilt rotten.

Mam disappears into the kitchen to make tea for Becky and coffee for me. The kettle must have been boiled in readiness, as it is only a few minutes before she returns with a tray loaded with steaming mugs and choc chip biscuits. Her warm smile only thinly disguises her habitual anxiety for her daughter, and I get the feeling that she is not at all sure what I am doing there, but I feel welcome nevertheless as she steers me towards an armchair close to the fire and makes sure that I am comfortable before conscientiously absenting herself. The china mug is hot in my hands and I put it carefully on the small table, conveniently placed by my chair, and sink into the softness of the plentiful cushions that mound up around me as I sit down. Becky carefully lets herself relax into an equally large collection of cushions at the end of the sofa opposite me and I can't help but notice the slowness in her movement, the slight wince of pain, as she does so. I notice too the obvious care she has taken with her appearance. Warmly dressed in a jumper and soft jersey trousers she looks as neat and as stylish as she did when we first met. Her hair, still short and as shockingly blonde, is beautifully cut and arranged so that it frames her carefully made-up face. Becky grins at me. She knows what I am thinking. She says, simply, 'I always try to look nice.'

We chat for a little while in the way that people do when they are building up to a more emotional conversation. She asks me about my journey and we talk about the weather and about how I have been since we last met. I begin to relax as the warmth of the fire seeps into me, and I ponder on how the room is spotless and as neat and tidy as Becky is herself. Furnished with obvious care and attention to detail, the neatness betrays the pride and determination with which she and her young husband have built their home around them, a young couple who have started out in life together looking forward as much as they can to a bright future. I tell her that her home is beautiful, 'Really welcoming', and Becky, although she is obviously pleased, allows her face to colour a little as she mutters something about the place being 'a mess'.

Beside her on the sofa there is a small pile of notebooks. I know that they contain her story, her experiences over the months since her first operation, all set down with honesty and conviction in her own words, her feelings translated into neat handwritten script. She started writing soon after the first *Drawing*

Women's Cancer exhibition at the Senedd, and a 'pain diary' suggested by her counsellor began to turn into something a lot more. All her emotions and all of the things that she cannot say to those who love her are in the notebooks. They contain between soft covers the narrative of her life and her loves, her pain and her passions. It is the narrative that she hopes, somehow, will help heal her and maybe, somehow, even help others heal too.

I notice that the books have become a little tattered over the months. Some of the covers are curling at the edges, but Becky sees me looking at them and, in what seems to be an almost unconscious movement, she puts out a protective hand and moves them aside. I pretend not to notice. There's no rush. I know that I need to let her tell me about the notebooks in her own time, so for now they lay, brooding on the sofa, until she is ready. I begin to tell her about what I have been doing with both *Drawing Women's Cancer* and the other medical projects I am working on, and although Becky responds politely she seems a little distracted, her attention more on the notebooks than on me. After a while she appears to make a decision, and, only a little self-consciously, she begins to tell me about how they came into being. 'I started writing in them after the exhibition... you said about how you were writing about us and I thought it was a good idea.'

I remember talking with her on that rain-soaked opening night. She was beautiful as she stood proudly amid the throng of people who, finally, wanted to talk with her about her illness, wanted to understand. She says, 'It was nice to speak with people who are in the same boat as myself or who know a lot about it... so you don't feel like you're in a corner. Like when you speak to people... a lot of people don't understand. When they said to me what it was... I didn't know... I'm not ashamed to say that I didn't know. Breast cancer isn't so embarrassing to speak about as something like this.'

Suddenly her smile fades a little. Her gaze drifts away again – not just from me this time but also from the room as a whole. Speaking quietly, as if to herself, she says that writing in the notebooks helps to 'get things straight in her head'. I say nothing. Indeed, there seems nothing of consequence *to* say. Becky does not need platitudes or sympathy. It is obvious that she continues to struggle with the physical and emotional consequences of both the original surgery and the several procedures she has undergone since, and it feels as if the most empathic thing I can do is say nothing and simply be with her. She looks at me directly and gifts me a rueful smile. 'I do have my low days.'

Two hours pass by as we talk, and it feels now as if our meeting is coming to a natural end. I can see that Becky is tired and in pain. It has taken no small amount of effort, both physically and emotionally, for her to bring the past back into focus. It is time to leave, but as I push my pad and pen into my bag, which is still damp from the rain, Becky suddenly and deliberately picks up her own pile of notebooks, saying, 'I never re-read what I write and I've never shown it to anybody, not even Matthew.' I nod, and she continues, 'I don't want anybody to read them until it's finished.' I nod again to show that I respect her wishes of course, even though I know inwardly that I would love to take a look at what she's written, and I ask, simply, '*Will* it finish?' Becky thinks for a moment.

'Perhaps when I have a baby.'

I smile, but as I get up to leave she suddenly makes a decision. She holds out the first of the pile, saying, 'Do you want a little read of them?' and I sit down again. I take the offered notebook and I feel the privilege weigh heavy on my shoulders as I read the first pages of fluent prose that speaks of ordinary things in an extraordinary way.

Becky's much-coveted normality is characterised in her written words, which tell of young love and young dreams, but it is in-between the lines that this normality becomes resonant of hope and defiance. Neither she nor I were to know then that the lines I read that day, together with the rest of her writing, would become the basis for the rest of Becky's story as it is narrated in the present book. A story told with unmitigated honesty and conviction, a story of raw and naked experience. But, on that day, there was one last thing I needed to ask before I left her warm and welcoming home, so, perhaps a little tentatively, I said, 'Is there a before and an after?' Becky looked up at me as if she had been half expecting the question but was still surprised that I had asked it. After a moment she answered, very quietly.

'No, I think it's more... it's just something that happened.'

I simply nodded, again. I wanted her to know then, and I hope that she knows now, that I understand.

SUTURE 2: Anita. Vulval Cancer

'Beyond myself'

Anita was diagnosed with vulval cancer in 2013. She had surgery twice that year, the first time in July, to remove the tumour, and again in October, to remove the surrounding lymph nodes. In December 2013 she suffered a blood clot in her heart. Anita agreed to talk with me after her follow-up appointment with her consultant and she seemed happy to tell me about her experiences of a life that includes the cancer as only one of many griefs.

She is a small woman, with dark hair and equally dark eyes that, despite her careworn expression, retain a mischievous sparkle. Slightly stooped, she moves with an obvious consciousness of her years as she takes her seat opposite me in the small, bare room at the women's clinic. Pulling her cardigan tighter around her shoulders, she makes herself as comfortable as she can in the hard, plastic chair and looks at me expectantly.

Feeling a little as if I am the one being interviewed, I begin by explaining a little about the project and I ask her permission to record the conversation. She agrees but still eyes the recorder with suspicion as she begins to tell me, in unabashed detail, about her experiences. Soon, however, as her story unfolds and she gets into her stride, she seems to completely forget its presence, even as it silently ensures her voice will remain in digital posterity.

> I had irritation, terrible irritation and I was scratching you know, and I felt something there. But I don't look you know, I'm not one to feel or prod. It was a long time before I went to the GP... When I did go he said it was a cyst, and when I did go to Dr T, *she* said it was a cyst. But when they took it away it was a cancer tumour! I had to come in and have

How to cite this book chapter:
Saorsa, J. with Phillips, R. 2019. *Like Any Other Woman: The Lived Experience of Gynaecological Cancer*. Pp. 41–45. Cardiff: Cardiff University Press.
DOI: https://doi.org/10.18573/book2.h. License: CC-BY-NC-ND 4.0

lymph nodes taken from the tops of both my legs and then I was ill for days. And then I had to go home with a vac pack. That was…

Anita had been talking increasingly fluently and quickly, but here she suddenly paused and stared at the floor as if there was something only she could see there. The memory of the operation and its aftermath was clearly a painful one. I simply wait, and make a mental note to find out exactly what a 'vac pack' is.

> A 'vac pack' is the colloquial name for equipment called a vacuum assisted wound closure kit. It is used in circumstances where it is necessary to drain excess lymph fluid from wounds where lymph glands have been removed. The vac pack consists of a drainage tube that is inserted into the wound and attached to a small portable vacuum pump and a container for the drained fluid. Once the tube is inserted, clips or a few stitches can be used to effect closure of the skin and a protective covering called Opsite, a cling film like dressing material, is then stretched over the wound. The aim is to create a sealed, airtight dressing so that excess fluid can be vacuum pumped away from the wound and disposed of. In cases where wound is large, or 'broken down', it may be 'packed' with gauze, or even with polyurethane foam, before the Opsite is applied but, because sometimes the seal can break, the vac pack kit is fitted with an alarm attachment, and this sends out a beeping sound as soon as any failure of the seal occurs.

After a few moments Anita seems to 'come back'. She looks up at me and says, 'I've never been so frightened.' Instinctively, I suppose – I certainly didn't think about it – I reach out and take her small hand in mine. Anita looks surprised, but she wraps her bony fingers around my palm and takes a deep breath before she suddenly leans towards me, almost conspiratorially, and says, 'I can't cope with anything to do with medical stuff or blood… I'm awful squeamish.'

Her memories of being diagnosed with vulval cancer are coloured by the shock and fear she says that she felt then and indeed still feels now when she thinks about it. But the emotions, she says, were not immediate. They came a little after the precise moment that the doctor told her. Her description of that moment stays with me, and even now, as I write, its emotive power affects me deeply, perhaps because it is derived from its simplicity. 'I went numb. My daughter was with me and she just fell apart, but I couldn't do anything. I went numb. I was beyond myself.'

There is another pause and, as her hand slips out of mine, I feel as if Anita has left me and has gone to that very place, beyond herself, that she evokes. The room feels colder, darker, as if the shadows have become a veil over the harshness of her memories. Then, in a softer, quieter, and this time slightly hesitant voice, she tells me about how, after the operations, she wouldn't, couldn't, look at herself. The sight of the scars on her body repulsed her, as they still do, and when she became very ill after the lymphadenectomy surgery it only compounded her misery. She admits that she isolated herself from her friends and even from her family and nursed her anger, her grief, alone.

There is a pervading feeling of regret in the room, and it takes over us both. I am caught up in her emotions. And indeed, we are caught up together as she describes how badly she feels she treated those around her while she was ill. She is close to tears, and I sense she has cried a lot over the years, but tears have never helped wash away the guilt that she is still harbouring for what she was when she became 'somebody else'. 'I was beyond myself, beyond myself.' She repeats the self-accusation almost like a chant, a chant for forgiveness, maybe, if only she could forgive herself. It reminds me of the first line of a Buddhist chant somebody once taught me. It seems so appropriate now.

May I be free of suffering. May I be at peace. May I be well.

But Anita is now looking directly at me. 'I was not myself,' she says with conviction.

> It was like it was happening to someone else. I had two district nurses come round every day to change the vac pack and dress it but the alarm would go off. If anything went wrong with it the alarm would go off and I'd be crying on the phone to my son and to my daughter and then the beep-beep would go off to say the seal had gone. I wasn't very good. I wasn't very confident in myself. I was a weak patient. I'd only just buried my brother a couple of months back – cancer – and I buried my other brother eight years ago. He had cancer too. I've got two sisters and when I knew it was cancer it was devastating. I don't think I'm a strong person. I didn't cope. No, I didn't.

'Weak patient' or not, Anita has clearly managed to cope with devastating medical problems over the past couple of years and, as I listen carefully to the story that she is telling me now in a much more animated way, I find out more about her life and I come to see a younger Anita in my mind's eye. I see the Anita who has had the strength and sense of purpose to raise four children single-handedly over 42 years after the shock of early widowhood; the Anita who has had to live through the pain of losing one of her sons, who died, suddenly, during a trip to Canada; the Anita who has buried two brothers. Her grief is palpable, but her resolve endures. No, this is not a weak woman sitting in front of me. This is a woman who has had to suffer more than her fair share of loss and heartache.

Anita draws breath and lapses once again into silence. In the effort of talking about her past her thoughts seem to have fallen around her like the leaves fall from a tree as the winter creeps in. I wait. The space her silence has created between us is not uncomfortable, and after a while she seems to gather up her leaves and hold onto them tightly in her small hands that are now bunched into fists in her lap. She begins again to tell me about what it felt like after the operation, how she had stayed in the house for fear of the world at large, while at the same time berating herself for being reliant on others. She tells me about a trip

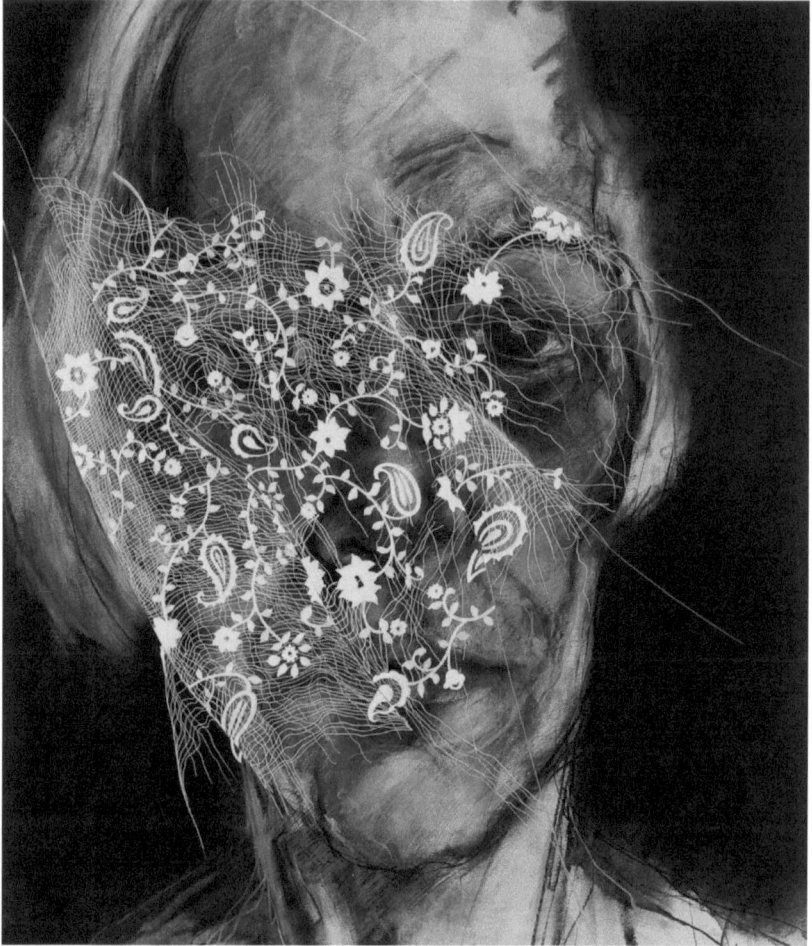

BEYOND MYSELF: *chalk, charcoal and white ink on paper*

This piece is inspired by the phrase Anita used to describe her reaction to her diagnosis. I drew in the fragment of lacy veil over the face in order to emphasise the feeling of being separated, suddenly, from all the woman had come to understand as normal life.

to Asda, with her son, just to do some shopping. Things went badly wrong. She had 'frozen'. The effort of containing all the anxieties that came with being in an environment other than home, where it felt safe, was too much, and she stood, rigid, gripping the handle of the shopping trolley until her knuckles whitened. Her son had been understanding, reassuring. He had brought her home, made her tea, but Anita's sense of shame over her vulnerability still eats away at her, even now, penance as she sees it for relinquishing herself to medical intervention, to giving up her autonomy, for becoming a patient, a burden.

I listen and I want to help her. I want to tell her that her reactions to what happened were natural, fundamentally understandable, and that her feelings of guilt and shame that they now give rise to are unwarranted. But I can't. My purpose here is not to placate, or pacify, or offer therapy. I must simply listen and allow Anita the space and time to say what she needs to say and to feel what she needs to feel. But I can hold her, metaphorically. I can offer her a safe space within the confines of empathy and respect. Suddenly she looks directly at me. She is smiling as she says, 'But things are better now!' Her voice sounds different, stronger, and as all the shadows dissipate I catch again that sparkle in her eye as she shifts in her chair, straightens up and seems to take command of herself. It is as if she has physically raised herself up from the emotional pit and she laughs gently and with self-deprecation as she tells me that she had lost over a stone in weight during her illness, but now she is putting the weight back on. She is worried now about becoming obese! It is a genuine concern, although clearly, from my detached perspective, an irrelevant one. She is certainly not overweight. Nevertheless, because she is so very excited about going to Yorkshire soon, to attend her daughter's wedding, she naturally wants to look her best. She leans forward again and, adopting that conspiratorial tone, she lets me know that she will buy her dress and hat when she gets to Yorkshire because, as she says with a wink of her eye, 'They have better shops up there.'

The conversation is coming to a natural end, and as I smile at Anita and she smiles back I see three aspects of her being, all concentrated into one small, yet very real and unique woman: the Self before, the ill Self and the Self after. All these selves make up the true Anita, the whole person with all her faults and all her indiscretions along with, and most importantly, all her wonderful kindnesses and strength and individuality. I'm not sure of course that Anita would agree with this assessment of her character, but either way I need to ask one last question before she leaves, so I take my courage in my hands.

'Can you forget?'

Anita hesitates, a worried frown crosses her face and I hope that by asking such a question I've not damaged her trust in me. Then she replies, with a raw and searing honesty,

'I want to say yes. But I don't know.'

She takes my hand to say goodbye and squeezes it tightly in hers. There is no need to say anything more.

Life is short, the Art long,
opportunity fleeting,
experience treacherous,
judgment difficult.

Hippocrates

Becky. Return Visit: Part 2

In writing it all down in her notebooks, both about her experiences with the cancer itself and about how her relationship with Matthew has grown through it all into the loving partnership they now share, Becky says that she has been able to find some release, even when it is too emotionally difficult for her to talk things through with her family and friends. Vulval cancer is not the sort of subject you raise easily in conversation, especially when you are trying, as Becky always is, to protect those she loves. For that first exhibition we produced a short annotated catalogue that alongside pictures of the artwork included information about vulval disease and direct quotes from the women I had worked with during the project to date. Becky tells me about how she was inspired by it and how she showed it to her relatives, especially to the male members of her extended family. She says that it 'worked' and that now they understand better. 'It was better for them to read it rather than have to explain everything to them. Then they didn't have to ask any questions.'

The impact of the cancer has been massive for Becky, physically, emotionally and socially. It has been a third party in her relationship, the monster in the room with her and Matthew, even in the beautiful new house they have bought together and made a home. In her story, however, diligently written down in fluent recollection, back in 2007 nobody had, as yet, given the monster its true name.

It was the day of my appointment and I was so glad I was seeing the nurse. I knew her quite well so I wouldn't find it so hard explaining things to her. We went into the room and I told her about the problems I was having during intercourse and about the lump in my groin and the colour of my skin. She asked me to get undressed and get up on the couch so she could have a look. She asked me if the lump was sore and I told her only sometimes. It all depends what underwear I wear. She also had a look at the colour of my skin but she told me it wasn't anything to worry about. When

How to cite this book chapter:
Saorsa, J. with Phillips, R. 2019. *Like Any Other Woman: The Lived Experience of Gynaecological Cancer.* Pp. 47–48. Cardiff: Cardiff University Press.
DOI: https://doi.org/10.18573/book2.i. License: CC-BY-NC-ND 4.0

I asked her about the pain I was getting during sex she told me that I need to relax more because I seemed to be tensing myself up too much, so in so many words I'm doing it to myself! I walked out of the room to meet my mother in the waiting area and I told her everything. She and I were glad there was nothing to worry about. I was so relaxed and happy. I was thinking to myself, 'It's OK. I'm like any other woman. I'm completely normal.'

But it wasn't OK. The lump she had in her groin and the discolouration of her skin turned out to be anything but normal.

Scars are tattoos with better stories.

Anonymous

SUTURE 3: The Survivors Group

Very early on in the *Drawing Women's Cancer* project, while we were waiting for the result of our application for ethical approval, I took advantage of an invitation to attend the first South East Wales Gynaeco-logical Oncology Centre Survivorship Event. I thought that it would be a good way to introduce myself to some of the medical staff I would no doubt be working with, and also an opportunity to get some idea of the sort of resources available for cancer patients.

As I arrive at the venue I have never been so unsure of what to expect, so I try to expect nothing. It is a very plush hotel where the staff always smile at you but never really see you, and the décor struggles to find its raison d'être between the personal and the impersonal, business and pleasure. I find my way to the second floor and the room where the event is to take place. It is already full of people. This event is shrouded in the personal, powerfully so, and as I enter the room I feel as though I am being drawn into the folds. Nevertheless, as I look around, trying to orientate myself in the crowd, I feel out of place. I am an outsider, and I feel as if I have gatecrashed the party of a small yet very exclusive club.

Everybody is friendly towards me, but despite their welcoming demeanour they still know the rules better than I do. A woman in a nurse's uniform stops me at the door and lets me know that I must not talk (officially) to the ladies who are cancer patients at all and that I can converse only with the nurses, medical staff and people manning the charity stalls. The nurse smiles sympa-thetically as she says, 'I'm sorry, but we've been told that you don't have the DBS check through yet.' Despite my limited remit, the enthusiasm of my welcome is tangible in the handshakes, the smiles, the offers of tea and cakes, but what am I doing here? What am I thinking in trying to organise this project? How will women who have suffered, who are suffering, and people who are caring for the

How to cite this book chapter:
Saorsa, J. with Phillips, R. 2019. *Like Any Other Woman: The Lived Experience of Gynaecological Cancer*. Pp. 51–54. Cardiff: Cardiff University Press.
DOI: https://doi.org/10.18573/book2.j. License: CC-BY-NC-ND 4.0

suffering, receive me, an artist, in the midst of perhaps the hardest of times in their lives? How will they respond to what I am trying to do?

Questions are unceasing in my head. They become impossible to control and impossible to answer as I gaze around the room. What of the disease and what of the person? What is and what becomes and/or remains the difference? What do outsiders, like me, see first? I am conscious that I am searching the crowd, trying to decide whether she has cancer, whether she is a nurse, whether she is a carer, and for whom? Everybody here has some connection to cancer, to gynaecological cancer, but who are the nurses, the surgeons, the charity workers? Everybody has their own unique reason for being here, but at the same time they are all here for one thing, to celebrate survivorship. They are so many strangers, but they are together, and with togetherness comes the freedom and security with which they are able to talk about something that, outside this room, is never so giving. Cancer is no longer the elephant in the room. *I* am.

People are moving towards the lines of chairs in the middle of the room and an audience is forming as the speakers are about begin. I find a chair near the back, beside an elderly lady. Even though she is seated I can tell that she is tall, and her features are delicate and refined. She is dressed expensively, impeccably, and her long, slim fingers gently clasp the strap of a small leather handbag that she holds in her lap. She does seem frail, and she has an air of vulnerability about her, but she smiles serenely at me as I ask politely if the seat beside her is free. She continues to smile as I sit down and she seems so very kind, so very interested in me. I know she thinks I am a fellow sufferer and I do indeed suffer, guilty for not correcting her, but I do not, cannot say, 'I am only an artist', not to the elderly lady who is so calm, so beautiful. I cannot explain it even to myself, but I feel as if admitting my healthy status would be almost like offering an insult.

The elderly lady's companion is a Zambian cleric. She tells me, in a soft whispery voice that sounds like water running over silk, that he is in contact with the wife of the Zambian president and that she, the president's lovely wife, is so very involved in cancer care. Here in this room, with a view through the huge plate glass windows that extends wide over the city, the idea of cancer care in Zambia, women with cancer, living and dying a continent away, seems strange. But in the beautiful lady's eyes, in her heart, it is clear that they are so very close. Where survivorship has the power to unite, the beautiful lady and her quiet, smiling companion speak loudly in its service, and yet, she also seems so unutterably sad. There is a shadow behind her smile that wreathes her hurt, hides her wounds. The beautiful lady has no time for the earnest complementary therapies speaker who begins the proceedings. It never shows in her serene expression but her slight body stiffens. She turns aside, still smiling, but she will not listen.

The second speaker is Rachel, aged 44 and recovering from vulval cancer. The beautiful lady is listening again but visibly flinching as the force of Rachel's passion makes hailstones of her words. Rachel is very 'active', a purposeful

campaigner who began fundraising even from her hospital bed. She talks eloquently, ardently, about the 'speakable', while she refers more quietly, more rev-
erently, to the 'unspeakable'. But everybody hears her. Everybody understands.
The beautiful lady understands. Her hands flutter in her lap and she turns to
smile at me again, warmly.

Every one of the speakers in turn refers to the ubiquitous idea of the 'cancer
journey', but I ask myself, where have they travelled to or from? Can the experience of cancer really be equated to a journey in itself? Or is it rather a complex
form of terminus, a possible end point situated along the route that we must
all take, whether healthy or sick, and from where some can simply journey on,
possibly in a different directions, and others cannot? More than this, how far
does this analogy of a journey, or any of the other common themes in its like,
go towards helping people cope with the actual experience of illness?

I am jolted out of my musings by Jenny, the hypnotherapist who has begun to
speak with utter and unabashed conviction. Indeed, she is almost evangelical
in her ideas about personal survivorship, and now she is exhorting the positive benefits of her 'thought management process'. 'This is not counselling,' she
enthuses. 'It is simply a way to let go of the negative molecules that lurk within
our memories.' Her own cancer 'journey', through double breast cancer and
endometrial disease, became, for her, a positive one. 'It made me realise why I
am here,' she says. 'I know now what I am here to do.' Now she is free of cancer
herself she encourages people to come to her to learn about thought management, and she lets us know, with no lack of pride in her own selfless concern for
others, that she does all this 'for free'.

Next the Macmillan welfare advisor takes the baton. She is here to help too.
When cancer causes your life to fall apart, when you have worries about your
job, your mortgage, your loss of earnings, the cost of your medicines, she is here
to advise. 'There are so many ways to help,' she says, and help certainly does
seem to be a permanent resident in cancer's domain. Help is always around the
corner on the cancer journey.

Next up, Nicky tells us all about the Butterfly House which her organisation wants to build because, on the journey, 'we all need somewhere to go'. Her
organisation needs to raise the money but she is confident that the House will
soon be standing. 'We have the architect's plans,' she says, proudly, and there is
a fierce defiance in her expression.

After the talks I chat with some of the nurses and I feel, with almost painful
relief, their polite scepticism turning slowly to interest, and to acceptance even,
but I still feel like an outsider, a trespasser, a stranger travelling through forbid-
den territory. I tell a nurse about who I am and what I am doing, my history, my
experience, my counselling training. And I tell her, 'I have had a hysterectomy
myself.' For a moment she looks at me as if unsure, but then she seems to come
to a decision. 'It's so exciting!' she says, and clasps my hand in hers.

I talk with a surgeon. He is a consummate professional and so very accommodating. 'Raise awareness,' he tells me. 'Do you know that people are just not

aware?' I do. I feel better. I talk with another nurse. 'Is it just cancer?' she asks. 'I know nurses who... lost children, childbirth, drug addiction, all sorts of things, all about women. Is it just cancer?' It is becoming overwhelming. Things are moving fast. So much interest now, and so many questions. 'You work with Dr T? She told us/called me/emailed me.' 'It seems so exciting.' 'With your background you seem perfect.' 'It's about the person.' 'It would be so good to have something to show the ladies that isn't so terrifying.'

The ladies themselves are queuing for tea donated by Twining's. There are homemade cupcakes too. The ladies are with their carers, husbands, friends. I am not sure what to do or who to be; it is hard to be myself.

Jenny says, 'Nobody talks about death.'

Somebody says, 'Nobody talks about down there.'

As I leave the meeting I am struggling to balance so many thoughts with so many feelings, but I know that all of them will turn into memories scribbled into my notebook and relived as I draw out the images in my head onto paper. And the memories will be positive, productive, devoid of 'negative molecules'.

When we love, we always strive to become bet-
ter than we are. When we strive to become better than
we are, everything around us becomes better too.

Paulo Coelho

Becky. Return Visit: Part 3

Becky was to wait some time before eventually it was discovered that the lump in her groin and the discolouration of her skin were actually far from normal, and during that time she had a lot to cope with, some good, some bad. Some of the good was very special, such as when, during the 2007 Christmas holidays, Matthew finally asked her to marry him.

> *Driving down over this little humpback bridge Matthew stops the car. He gets out, walks around to my side, opens the car door and goes down on one knee. He finally pops the question! It was raining quite heavy and he was trying to be so serious but the things he said to me were so beautiful it was really romantic. I couldn't have asked for anything better.*

She was elated. During the year there had been two weddings in the family and Becky had been bridesmaid, but now she and Matthew were beginning to plan their own 'big day'. For Becky this was everything she had wanted. They set the date: 25 September 2010. 'Plenty of time to prepare', and, besides, they had house-hunting on their minds. The search began in the New Year, and in the summer of 2008:

> *We spotted a house we both liked that had a for sale sign on it and I was real cheeky, I knocked on the door and asked the owner how much the house up was up for sale for. She invited me in and showed me around. She was lovely. It was perfect really and because it was the start of our summer everything looked so light and fresh. I managed to get an official viewing the following day and I asked my mother to come with us. It doesn't matter how old I am, I always ask my parents opinion. We liked everything we saw and when I looked at Matthew and I could see by his face how much he liked it. My mother thought it was beautiful. We put*

How to cite this book chapter:
Saorsa, J. with Phillips, R. 2019. *Like Any Other Woman: The Lived Experience of Gynaecological Cancer.* Pp. 57–62. Cardiff: Cardiff University Press.
DOI: https://doi.org/10.18573/book2.k. License: CC-BY-NC-ND 4.0

in an offer and they accepted it! As we were waiting for everything to go through we were doing as much shopping as we could to make sure everything was in place ready for when we had the keys. Everything was coming together nicely. I got myself a new job and I was only ten minutes down the road from the house. We were so excited. The solicitor told us we should have the keys by early September so I arranged for all our furniture to get delivered but unfortunately we didn't get the keys when we should have so I had to rearrange all the deliveries. Eventually we had the keys on the 27th September, which was my birthday!

Despite the good times there were, as there always are in life, things that were not quite so happy, things that drew heavily on Becky's emotional reserves. In quick succession three members of her family, all of whom she loves with a bottomless depth of feeling, suffered sudden assaults on their health. Her father became seriously ill and was hospitalised. Her grandmother, a fundamental figure in Becky's life, died, and her husband-to-be, Matthew, had to undergo extensive surgery for a severe back injury. Her father recovered well but Matthew had continuing problems, which left him debilitated and dependent for a long time. In the midst of all this, Becky's own health issues were almost forgotten, that is until she received the results of a routine smear test.

I never really worried about my smear results and anyway I couldn't really fit that bit in my brain, there was enough going on in there as it was with Matthews back being so bad and seeming to get worse. We didn't know what the next step was going to be. He would go to physio on a regular basis every week but it wasn't helping and money was getting tight. Weeks passed and there was no signs of the steroid injections working on Matthews back. I also received my smear results through the post. It said that my results had come back abnormal so I had to phone my doctors to have another one done. I knew Mam had had the same problem for years. She would have one normal smear and then an abnormal one and it went on like that for some time. Perhaps it was going to be the same with me. Matthew had to stop going to physio because it was making his back worse. It had been a few months now since he had to come out of work but we had started getting used to handling what money we had. We were thinking about having a dog.

The treatment you need for abnormal cervical cell changes depends on whether you have mild, moderate or severe changes. Many women with mild changes don't need treatment as the changes go back to normal on their own. (Cancer Research UK)

Charlie settled in great. He was really good because after only about two weeks he would ask to go out for a wee. I was back to work as usual but with Matthew and Charlie in the house, some days I didn't feel like going at all. During that week Matthew rang me in work to tell me my second set of smear results had come back. The first thing I thought to myself was 'God they came back quick'. The results were abnormal again and now I was starting to worry. I had to go to the Royal Glamorgan hospital for a biopsy. I didn't have to wait long at all for an appointment. I told myself that everything was going to be fine.

If you have an abnormal screening test result you might have a referral to the colposcopy clinic for a closer look at your cervix. During this examination, your doctor or specialist nurse (colposcopist) can take samples (biopsies) of any abnormal areas. (Cancer Research UK)

Matthew came for the ride to the hospital but he waited in the car, what with him not being able to walk that far. Mam came in with me. When we were sitting in the waiting area I saw so many posters on the walls with different things like cancers, babies, and some of the things were quite worrying. When the nurse called me I thought my Mam could come in with me but she couldn't, I really wanted her there but she wasn't allowed. When I walked into the room the doctor who was going to do the biopsy was sitting there and I nearly died when I saw he was a man. He shook my hand and introduced himself. His name was Dr W and even though he was a man he was extremely nice. He made me feel very comfortable. I had to get onto the couch and lie back with my legs up in stirrups so that he could take the biopsy and I am not going to lie, it was quite painful. I was thinking to myself, 'He hasn't mentioned anything about the lump in my groin or the discolouration in my skin so it must be OK.' It was all done. It didn't take that long and then the doctor explained to me what would happen next. He said the results would be back in two to four week's time. I was so glad that I had that day off work because I had such a bad belly after the appointment.

There are a few different treatments that can remove the area of abnormal cervical cells. The advantage of these treatments is that the piece of cervical tissue that the colposcopist removes can be sent for examination under a microscope. In the laboratory, the pathologist rechecks the level of cell changes in the piece of tissue to make sure your screening result was accurate. They also closely examine the whole piece of tissue to make sure that the area containing the abnormal cells has been completely removed. (Cancer Research UK)

Matthew seemed to be picking himself up a little, especially with Charlie around for company. The old Matthew was coming back again and it was such a relief. We love each other deeply. We are there for each other and we laugh together, but to be honest we are incredibly childish. What's the point

*in being serious and grown up all the time? That isn't us. I never used to
believe it when older people say 'I still feel twenty one in the head', but I do
understand it now because I don't think I will ever feel my age.*

*My results for the biopsy came back still abnormal and I had to ring the
hospital to make an appointment because the letter said that I was to have
laser treatment done. I rang the hospital straight away but I asked if could
I have the appointment on a Monday, my day off, because it just makes it
easier if I don't have to worry about work. That was no problem, I had to
wait two weeks but that was fine with me. I could tell that Matthew was
really worried about me but he wouldn't say too much or ask any questions because he didn't want to worry me as well. Instead, he would ask
my mother.*

Laser therapy is sometimes called laser ablation. This just means the laser burns
away the abnormal cells. You have this treatment as an outpatient. A laser beam
is a very strong, hot beam of light. It burns away the abnormal area. You may
notice a slight burning smell during the treatment. This is nothing to worry
about. It is just the laser working. You can go home as soon as this treatment is
over. (Cancer Research UK)

*On the morning of my appointment I had planned to go to the hospi-
tal and then go and do some food shopping so I was really hoping that
I wouldn't have a bad belly like I had the last time. It wasn't as bad as I
thought it was going to be though, the treatment only took half an hour.
Dr W told me that I could have some bleeding and I was to have no sex for
at least two weeks. He said I should return to the hospital in six months
time for another routine smear. The pain after the laser treatment wasn't
too bad at all. I took painkillers all day to make sure it wouldn't get a hold
on me and after a few hours it seemed to settle down. Now it was all over
and there was nothing to worry about I got back to sorting out as much as
I could for our wedding.*

The term 'vulva' refers to a woman's external sex organs, including the skin surrounding them. It is made up of the opening of her vagina, which is surrounded
by two pairs of lips, or labia. The inner pair is called the labia minora and the
outer pair is called the labia majora. Just above the opening of a woman's vagina
is the opening of her urethra, a tube that runs from the bladder and through
which she passes urine out of her body. Her clitoris, the female sexual organ,
is located just above the urethra. In the majority of cases of vulval cancer the
tumour initially develops in one of the labia.

*We went to a lot a wedding Fayres so that we could get some ideas about
what we wanted. We had eighteen months to prepare and it really didn't*

seem that long at all. The biggest things were all sorted early on but it was the little things that were important like favours, centrepieces, the invitations and, of course, our wedding rings. By Christmas 2009 we had a lot sorted and ready for the wedding but we still needed the invitations. I wanted to make them myself. I wanted to make them personal to us. I came up with the idea of white invitations with a silver border and silver bow, with a photograph of me and Matthew when we were both three years old. Underneath the caption would be, 'Today I will marry my best friend.' Then there was the dreaded table planner. It was the hardest thing to do and it took weeks to get it right. I would start it, then scrap it and stat it again many times before it was finally done. But things seemed to be getting back on track as much as they could I suppose. The dog and the wedding were keeping Matthews mind occupied. The Stag and Hen do's needed sorting and us girls booked a weekend in Magaluf. Matthew didn't want to go away for a weekend because of his back so he decided on a day at the races. Now we were really starting to get excited.

The symptoms of vulval cancer may include a noticeable lump, mass or wart-like growth on the vulva, a persistent itchy sensation, pain or bleeding when passing urine, or a bloody discharge.

It was almost time for my follow-up smear at the hospital and even though my laser treatment was a success the lump in my groin was still annoying me so I decided that when I went for the smear I'd ask the doctor about it. On the day of my appointment, when I told Dr W why I wanted to see him and showed him the lump he couldn't understand why he didn't see it when I had the laser treatment done and after he did the smear he took a biopsy of the lump. He said I would have to wait around six weeks for my results. There was a worried look on my mothers face and I tried to explain it all to her, and to Matthew, but it was hard because, to be honest, I was worried too. I really hadn't been feeling right but I didn't know what was wrong. I put it down to being tired.

Later that week while I was having a bath I noticed a few red spots on the inside of my left leg. They were really sore. I went to bed that night feeling rotten and I felt no better when I woke up. I really didn't feel well enough to go to work but I went anyway and by the end of the day I could hardly put my legs together because it was just too sore. It was too late to go to my GP so I phoned the out of hours number, as I really wanted to see someone. They gave me an appointment for later that evening at the hospital near my Mothers house. Mam said she would come with me. I had shingles! No wonder that I was feeling so ill. I stayed on the couch that night with my feet up. Mam was panicking because I wasn't well and she wasn't happy.

By the end of the week I was feeling a lot better and I was able to return to work. I thought that all of the shingles had gone but about a week later I felt something again that was real sore. I had a look with a mirror and I noticed a red patch inside my vulva. I thought it must be a shingle but it was strange for it to still be there when all the rest were gone. I phoned Mam and she wanted me to make an appointment with the doctor so the following day, in my lunch hour, I rang my GP and the nurse, Louise, answered the phone. She told me to go straight to the surgery after work.

Vulval cancer mainly affects older women over the age of 65, and many of these women will have had a history of non-cancerous skin conditions affecting their vulva. The most common of these conditions is lichen sclerosus, which causes itchy white patches on the genitals. There is no cure for lichen sclerosus but treatment, including surgery, may bring some relief and prevent the condition escalating into vulval cancer.

Louise had a look at the red spot but she wasn't sure what it was so she called one of the doctors in. But the doctor wasn't sure either, so they referred me to a dermatologist. I still hadn't got my results from the previous test and all this waiting was starting to pick away at me. Eventually, on a Tuesday afternoon the phone rang at work and it was my Dad saying that the hospital had phoned but they wouldn't tell him anything. He gave me the number and I spoke to Dr W's secretary. She told me that my results were back and I was booked in to go to theatre the following day at 12.30pm. She couldn't tell me anything else. I couldn't hold back the tears because I didn't know what was going on.

It was a tense twenty-four hours. I had to be in the hospital by 7.30am and Matthew and my Mam were coming with me. We waited for a few hours and none of us really spoke. We didn't know what to say. In the end Dr W walked into the room to explain to me why I was there. He said that the biopsy results for the lump in my groin had come back pre-cancerous.

SUTURE 4: How Do You Know How Much to Cut?

The word 'gynaecology' is rooted in the Greek, gynaika, meaning woman, and logia, meaning study. Quite literally, the study of women.

Valerie, waiting for her operation to remove abnormal cells, is very proud of the fact that she has volunteered to talk to me. She says that she is glad to be a part of the *Drawing Women's Cancer* project and very happy to be involved, 'If it helps'. Rosalind, waiting for her operation to partially remove her vulva, is also happy to be involved, 'If it helps'.

The word empathy derives from the German Einfühlung (from ein, meaning 'in' and Fühlung, meaning 'feeling'.) It was first introduced in 1858 by German philosopher Rudolf Lotze as a translation of the Greek empatheia, meaning 'passion' or 'state of emotion', and as a term to define a theory of art appreciation wherein engagement with the art object depends on the viewer's ability to project his personality into it.

Pre-op: Valerie: 82 years old. Lichen sclerosus. Procedure four years ago (2010) to remove abnormal cells. Present repeat procedure (2014)

Valerie smiles and even waves to the other patients as we leave the ward and follow Dr T, her consultant surgeon, to the 'quiet room', where we will be able to talk privately and undisturbed. Once in the corridor Valerie's smile fades. The brave face she puts on for her fellow patients is no longer needed and her

How to cite this book chapter:
Saorsa, J. with Phillips, R. 2019. *Like Any Other Woman: The Lived Experience of Gynaecological Cancer.* Pp. 63–68. Cardiff: Cardiff University Press.
DOI: https://doi.org/10.18573/book2.l. License: CC-BY-NC-ND 4.0

expression relaxes into a quiet resignation, with just the odd flicker of pain that causes her to wince and draw breath. She shuffles slowly alongside me, sliding her feet so that the soles of her soft, pale green slippers barely leave the tiled floor, and leaning heavily on my arm. In stark contrast, Dr T, tall and long-limbed in her blue surgical scrubs, lopes along ahead of us, setting an impossible pace. Her mind is perhaps on the operation she is to about to perform rather than on the speed at which Valerie, her patient, is able to move.

Pre-op: Rosalind: 73 years old. Recurrent vulval cancer. Present procedure (2014) full vulval excision

I meet with Rosalind for the first time on the ward. She lies quietly in bed, covers pulled up to her chin so that only her face is visible. Her deep-set eyes peer at me over narrow, sharp cheekbones and her face is bordered by wispy, greying hair. She is expecting me, greets me with a smile. I notice how her nose wrinkles upwards like a girl's, and her eyes seem to disappear as the smile broadens and softens her whole face. It affects me deeply to feel so welcome. Against my protestations Rosalind heaves herself up to a sitting position and pulls a thick woollen cardigan around her shoulders. She folds her hands onto her lap, expectant, eager to begin. Some of the other women on the ward look on with interest and I feel a little self-conscious. Rosalind notices them too and nods gratefully when I ask if she'd prefer to go to the 'quiet room' to talk. As she moves to get out of the bed a nurse approaches and asks, or rather demands, to know where she's going. I begin to explain but the nurse simply ignores me and continues to interrogate Rosalind, who answers, reluctantly, with a monosyllabic mutter. The nurse sighs, as if she is dealing with a recalcitrant child. 'Well.' Her voice is imperious and she is standing square with her hands on her hips. 'Just as long as we know where you are. You'll need to see the anaesthetist soon.' With that the nurse turns abruptly away, again taking no account of my existence, and fixes her attention on another patient. Rosalind, grinning now and with a mischievous glint in her eye, gives me a wink and asks me to bring her walking frame to the bedside. Once she's ready we move on.

...

Valerie and I finally make it to the quiet room and Dr T cheerfully takes her leave with a reassuring smile. I shut the door after her. Small and windowless, the room is sparsely furnished with a worn sofa, visibly sagging under a long history of use, and a slightly more comfortable-looking armchair. Between these, in the middle of the room, there is a small low table on which there are some tattered and very out-of-date magazines. The floor is covered with carpet, a little threadbare and of a dirty-grey, nondescript colour that does nothing to warm up the pale, clinically blue paint that covers the walls and, unusually, the ceiling too. Lighting is limited to the harsh glare of a fluorescent tube, which hums softly. This then is the place where things can be discussed in private. This is where patients can be with their loved ones, where doctors can give out good news or bad, where relief can revive the living and where tears can be shed for the dead. For all this, I feel it could be more welcoming, comforting, but the cold blue walls and the worn carpet is all we have and so I steer Valerie to the chair and, once she is settled, I risk the sofa. I sink so low into the battered cushions that it feels as if I'm on the floor. My knees are almost beside my ears. Valerie, now looking down at me, tries to be polite but in the end we both have to laugh at the absurdity of it.

...

Rosalind makes a beeline towards the armchair as we enter the 'quiet room'. 'If I sit in there,' she says, motioning towards the sofa, 'I will never get up!' Of course I already know what she means but it is still a little disconcerting when the worn and sagging cushion gives way almost to the floor as I sit down.

...

Valerie is a living, breathing statistic. I remember a young scientist working with VIN cell cultures, who told me that 'a lot of the ladies with VIN, they get recurrent disease. They go back, I read that some ladies go back three, maybe four times.' Valerie, at 82 years old and about to return to theatre after four years, is alone in a crowd.

...

Rosalind doesn't want to talk about what she's been going through; she prefers to begin by telling me about her grandson. He is just four years old, and the look on Rosalind's face and the softness in her tone as she tells me about him speak volumes about how much she dotes on him. She tells me how very sad she feels because she cannot play with him as she used to, because of her 'condition'. The 'real' pain here is not so much physical, not so much rooted in, or experienced through the condition itself; it is emotional. It is a pain caused by the complete overturning and disruption of normal family life, of expectations, of healthy hopes and of dreams. Rosalind's eyes are shining in the cold light of the room with tears that she can no longer brook. I instinctively reach out to take her hand for a second, just as there's a loud knock on the door.

A nurse I've not met before fixes me in the open doorway with a look of suspicion. Clearly nobody has let her know who I am or anything about what I'm doing, and she glances at Rosalind with something akin to concern as I try to explain. I feel oddly vulnerable, as if I've been doing something wrong, and Rosalind simply looks at the floor. The nurse is in a hurry; she seems flustered, harassed and clearly has no time to listen to what I am saying. She glares and almost barks at me. 'But who are you? And what do you mean, you are an artist?' I step back, hands up. I don't need this, not today, not in front of Rosalind.

...

Valerie begins by telling me how cold she feels in the hospital, and I worry about how she pulls her towelling robe tighter around herself. 'I had to get up three times in the night,' she says. 'Just to walk around, because I was so cold.' We talk about the weather in general and about the merits of duvets over hospital blankets. Valerie, seemingly grateful to have a willing listener, gets into her stride. 'They tuck the sheets in so tightly at the bottom. I had to bring my pillows half-way down the bed just to get the covers around my neck!' I am beginning to regret leaving my sweater in Dr T's office but I simply nod, smile, and follow Valerie where she leads so that as we talk it begins to feel as if the temperature in the room is rising with the level of trust. Valerie allows me to cross the threshold of her world as she tells me about her family, her sons, but I see after a while that her gaze is no longer on me but somewhere further away, somewhere in the middle distance. She says, 'I never had a sister. I wanted girls, but now I have four granddaughters.' Then she smiles, still looking past me, as if there was a window in the wall behind me and she could see her granddaughters playing outside.

...

The nurse calms down and mutters what I choose to hear as an apology. She has come because the anaesthetist is ready to see Rosalind. With a rueful smile Rosalind obediently shuffles out of the room, leaning heavily on her walking frame, and I fall back, and down once again, into the sofa. I begin to scribble some notes but my pen runs out and I feel suddenly very tired – exhausted, in fact. If I actually take a minute to think about it, I have to acknowledge that I am working on autopilot.

...

Valerie talks about the future for her grandchildren and her worry for them in a 'difficult world'. She seems sad but calm, even pragmatic. But it is as if she is not really here in this small, slightly depressing room, huddled in her robe. It seems too as if she is not really about to undergo a surgical procedure, the extent of which she will have no idea of until she wakes up. No, she is elsewhere, maybe in the garden, in the sunshine, playing with her granddaughters as she did when, some time ago, she never had to worry about abnormal cells. She gives a low, barely audible sigh and then comes back to me, smiling again as she tells me about her husband. He is older than her. He is coming to see her in the afternoon so that he doesn't have to drive after dark. She says that she hopes she will have come round from the operation by the time he arrives.

...

This place is efficient – no room it seems for feelings, for the emotional content of the patients' experience. The 'ladies' are simply 'on the list'. It's not that the professionals do not care, I hope. No, of course they do. It is more that they can't allow themselves to care too much. They have a job to do and whether the patients have grandchildren or elderly husbands is not on their minds, at least not as it is on Rosalind's and on Valerie's. The individual here is hidden within the crowd, humanity subjugated to a general overall regime of care, but how else could it be? And me? I am to be accommodated yet wondered at. But what is the import of me? Of my presence here? What do I mean, 'I am an artist'? So I sit, waiting in the quiet room as the ward bustles around the open door and snippets of conversation float in and out. Nurses and staff are chatting, laughing and going about their business as if the pain of Rosalind's yearning to play with her grandson, and Valerie's haunting fears of developing full blown cancer are not still hanging in the air. Yet, the emotions are pervasive and they weigh heavy on me. I feel weakened with the burden. I wonder if I have time to get a coffee before I attend Rosalind's operation. I take it black, strong.

...

Valerie and I reach a pause in the conversation. Not an impasse, not uncomfortable, just a hiatus, a space filled with trust and within which there is no necessity to say anything at all. I simply wait, and after a few moments Valerie begins to talk about her son's recent divorce. Her tone is disapproving as she tells me about the plans he has made. The light in the room suddenly flickers and we laugh, nervously. Valerie says, 'That doesn't bode well!' We laugh again.

...

Rosalind lies motionless and masked on the table. I have changed into scrubs, sketchbook and drawing pen in hand. Rosalind has been given a local anaesthetic and is under light sedation, just on the edge of consciousness for the sake of 'time'. This way her recovery time will be shorter and, besides, there is another patient on the surgeon's list today. I see concern – no, more than that, fear in Rosalind's face, and as the operation begins I wonder at the wisdom of the arrangement when she complains of feeling pain. But it's not pain from the cutting, more from the unnatural position of her pelvis, her legs pulled up and out with her feet secured in rubber stirrups. Exposed, she moves very slightly and the surgeon stops working for fear of cutting too far. From behind her mask she mutters, sotto voce, 'Please try to stop her moving.' The junior doctor beside her looks embarrassed, but she replies quietly and firmly, glancing quickly over the surgeon's head in my direction. 'It's the discomfort. She'll settle down.'

...

The mood changes with the light. I tell Valerie a little more about the project. She is polite, but I sense that it is a world too far away. For her, it is enough to know that she is doing something to help. She is in no hurry to know all the details, until, that is, I mention that part of the work is to address the need for more patient-centred information about her condition. She frowns, and her voice takes on an edge that I haven't heard before. 'The nurse gave me a booklet. It wasn't very good. Some of it was about lichen sclerosus but some of it was about vulval cancer! The nurse crossed out all the stuff about cancer but you could read it still! Then she gave me another book about cancer and she said, "You haven't got cancer but you might find this interesting!"'

...

Rosalind seems to lapse into sleep and the operation begins again, but after only a couple of minutes there is another interruption. The junior doctor has to leave. She has 'come all over queasy'. Stammering her apologies, she moves quickly to the door. 'I'm sorry... I've been ill... flu... sorry'. And then she was gone. There is room now for me to get closer, and I move to stand behind the surgeon, who is working from a stool at the end of the table, sitting between Rosalind's tortured legs. She discovers the cancer, a hard, spherical, white intrusion into pink, healthy tissue. The crab in its shell. It's the margins that pose the problem. Cut too little and the chances of recurrence are high; cut too much and the patient suffers unnecessarily. But the vulva is delicate, the tissue fragile; absolute precision becomes impossible in this situation, yet the surgeon now works quickly and efficiently, making no more remarks about the occasional movements of her patient. Afterwards, once she has finished up the paperwork, I ask a question that is burning in me.

'Are you happy with how that went?'

I am concerned, but I try not to sound accusative. So many questions jostle with each other in my mind and I do need to voice them at some point but, for now, this will be enough. The surgeon shrugs. There is a defeated look in her dark eyes.

'The potential for recurrence is high,' she says. 'But how do you ever know how much to cut away?'

I agree: how do you ever know how much to cut?

Becky. Return Visit: Part 4

Vulval cancer itself is rarely diagnosed in younger, pre-menopausal women, but the incidence in the UK has risen over recent years and especially in those with a history of infection with the human papilloma virus, or HPV. Cancer-causing types of HPV, specifically HPV16 and HPV18, are the primary cause of cervical cancer, and, as they also cause skin cells in the vulva to undergo pre-cancerous changes, they are also responsible for the majority of cases of vulval intraepithelial neoplasia, or VIN. Like lichen sclerosus, VIN carries within it the potential for vulval cancer.

> *It was a massive shock. I just wasn't expecting that. He said that I had to have the lump removed and he was going to take another biopsy of the sore patch I had inside my vulva area. After that things seemed to move pretty quick. I went to theatre and before I knew anything I was waking up in recovery. When I got to the ward Dr W was waiting beside my bed to explain a few things to me. Mam and Matthew weren't back yet as they'd thought the operation would take longer and to be honest I couldn't make any sense of what the doctor said because I was still drowsy and I couldn't concentrate on what he was telling me. When Matthew and my mother came back a nurse told Mam that Dr W wanted to speak with her. She was gone only for about twenty minutes but when she walked back onto the ward she looked like she had seen a ghost. She was very upset. The doctor had told her that there was a possibility that I could have vulval cancer and, if it was cancer, then the necessary operation would be very disfiguring for a young woman of my age.*

There are, in all, five forms of vulval cancer, each one classified according to the type of cell within which the cancer first develops. Vulval cancer is in itself a rare disease compared with other gynaecological cancers, and only two of the

How to cite this book chapter:
Saorsa, J. with Phillips, R. 2019. *Like Any Other Woman: The Lived Experience of Gynaecological Cancer.* Pp. 69–74. Cardiff: Cardiff University Press.
DOI: https://doi.org/10.18573/book2.m. License: CC-BY-NC-ND 4.0

five main forms are commonly encountered, the primary form being squamous cell carcinoma.

> *It was a lot for all of us to take in. Later that day, when I was discharged Dr W gave me an appointment for five days time to talk about my results. To make things worse, Matthew was due to go back into hospital himself that week to have another back operation, so that meant he wouldn't be able to come with me to my appointment. He was going to have to stay in for a week and me and Charlie would move back in with my parents until he came home. Them five days of waiting and worrying both about Matthew and about me were an absolute nightmare for all of us. I hardly slept at all. On the day of my appointment I was up early and ready to go.*

Squamous cell carcinoma accounts for over 90 per cent of vulval cancers. In this form the tumour, or lesion, develops in the outermost skin layers of the woman's vulva.

> *Me and Mam got to the hospital in good time only for the lady behind the desk to tell us Dr W was running an hour behind. I thought, 'Of all the days, why today?' We went to get a coffee and waited. The time dragged so slowly but a nurse finally called me into the room and I saw Dr W sitting there with another nurse standing behind. I knew it was bad news. He sat me down and said, 'I am terribly sorry, but it is cancer'.*

Becky's cancer was squamous cell carcinoma.

> *I froze. I didn't know what to say. My poor Mam was terrible, I really felt for her. It was awful seeing her like that, I just wanted it all to stop. Dr W told me was he was referring me to an oncologist at Llandough hospital. Her name was Dr T. I will always remember him telling me this type of thing was her 'bread and butter'.*

The prognosis for squamous cell carcinoma is good. A large percentage of women will survive for at least five years after diagnosis and, where the cancer is discovered in its early stages, many women will be completely cured.

> *I had to phone Matthew to tell him the bad news. He asked me if we were going to be OK and I made sure I reassured him. I had to be strong even though I felt like I was breaking inside. I rang work to tell Lindsey I wouldn't be going back. She was so upset, I just didn't know what to say to people to try and make it easier. For the next few days everything was a blur. I thought I was going to wake up from a bad dream, this couldn't be real, but it was so I just had to get on with it. I spent most of that week at the hospital with Matthew and after seven days he was allowed home. We*

still weren't really sure how the operation on his back had gone so it was fingers crossed. But we had our wedding to look forward to.

My appointment to arrange the operation was fast approaching and I was trying to prepare myself for what the oncologist might say. Meanwhile Matthew was recovering quite well after his own operation. I'd never heard of vulval cancer before so I had a little look on the Internet. I didn't read too much, I only wanted to understand what it was, but one thing I did read was it was extremely rare in young women and it normally it affects women between sixty and eighty years old.

Because of the extreme difficulty in ensuring that all of the cancer is cut away on this delicate part of a woman's body, surgery is often followed by chemotherapy and/or radiotherapy.

The oncologist was so nice she really made me feel comfortable. I trusted her. We went through everything and she explained how big the operation was going to be. It was a lot for all of us to take in. Dr T wanted me to meet the plastic surgeon Dr D, but he couldn't make it that week so I had to make an appointment for the following week. I already kind of knew what the operation was about but Dr T wanted to be a hundred per cent certain that Dr D agreed with how she wanted to do it.

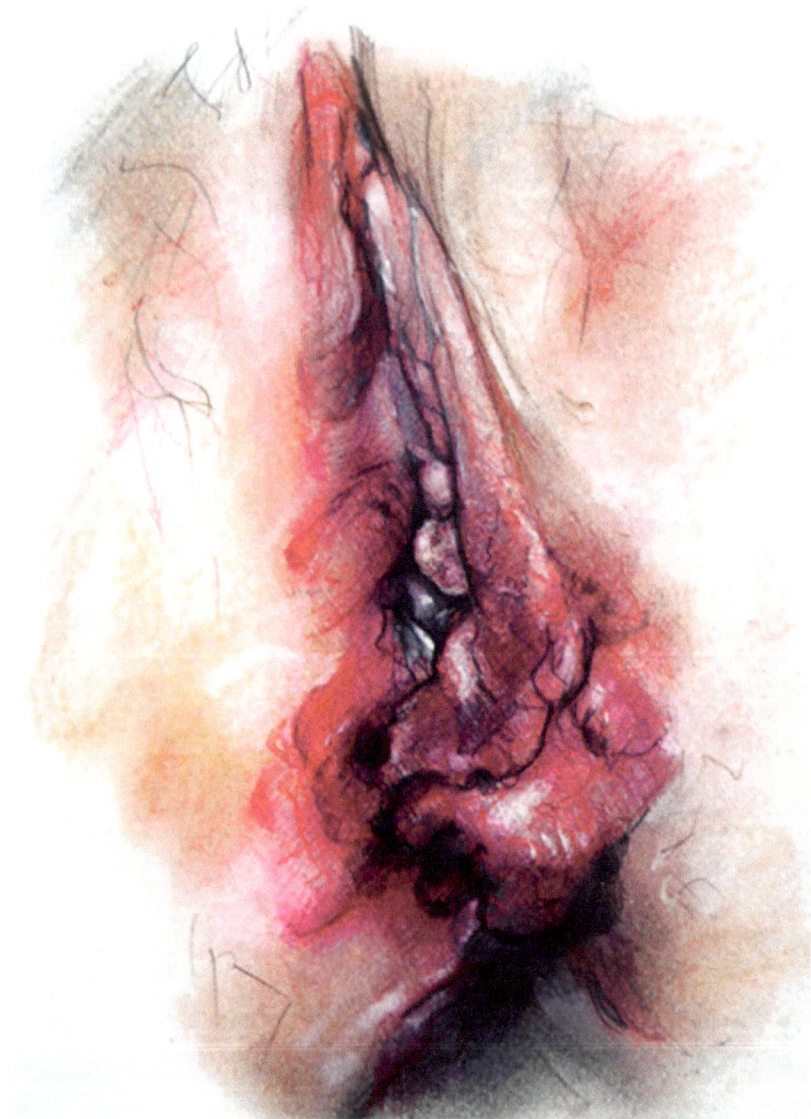

VULVAL CANCER BEFORE SURGERY: *coloured pencil on paper*

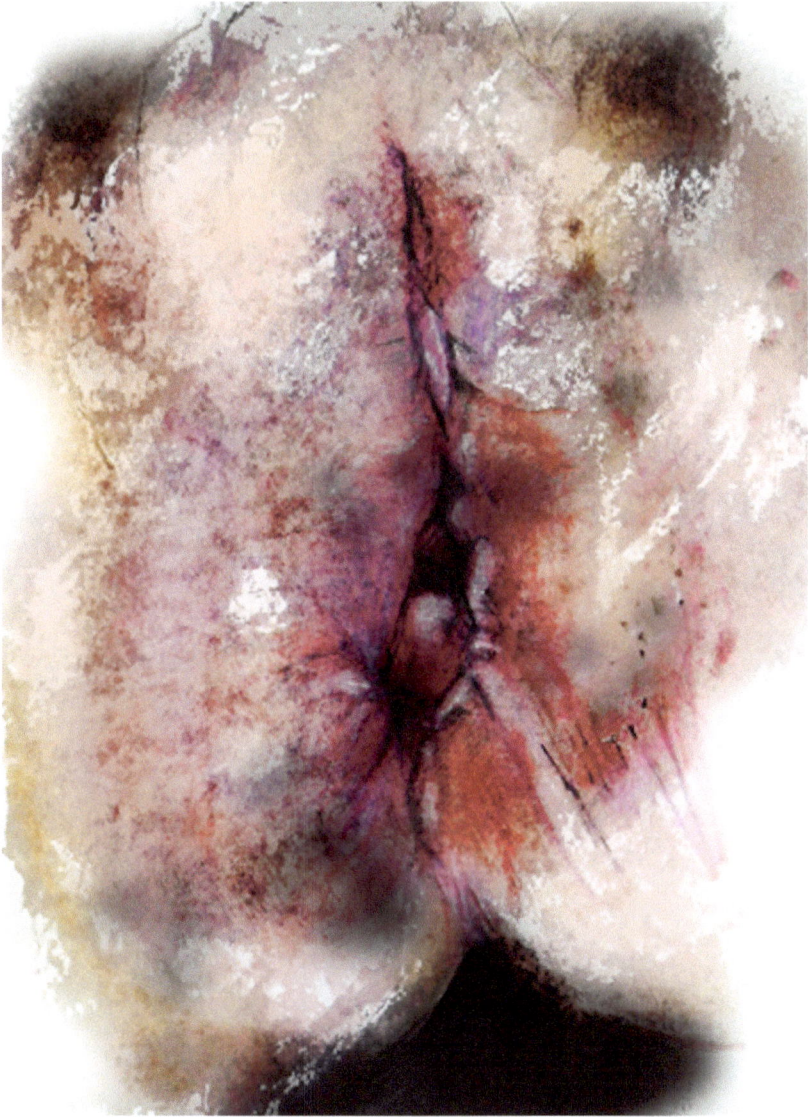

VULVA DIRECTLY AFTER SURGERY: *coloured pencil on paper*

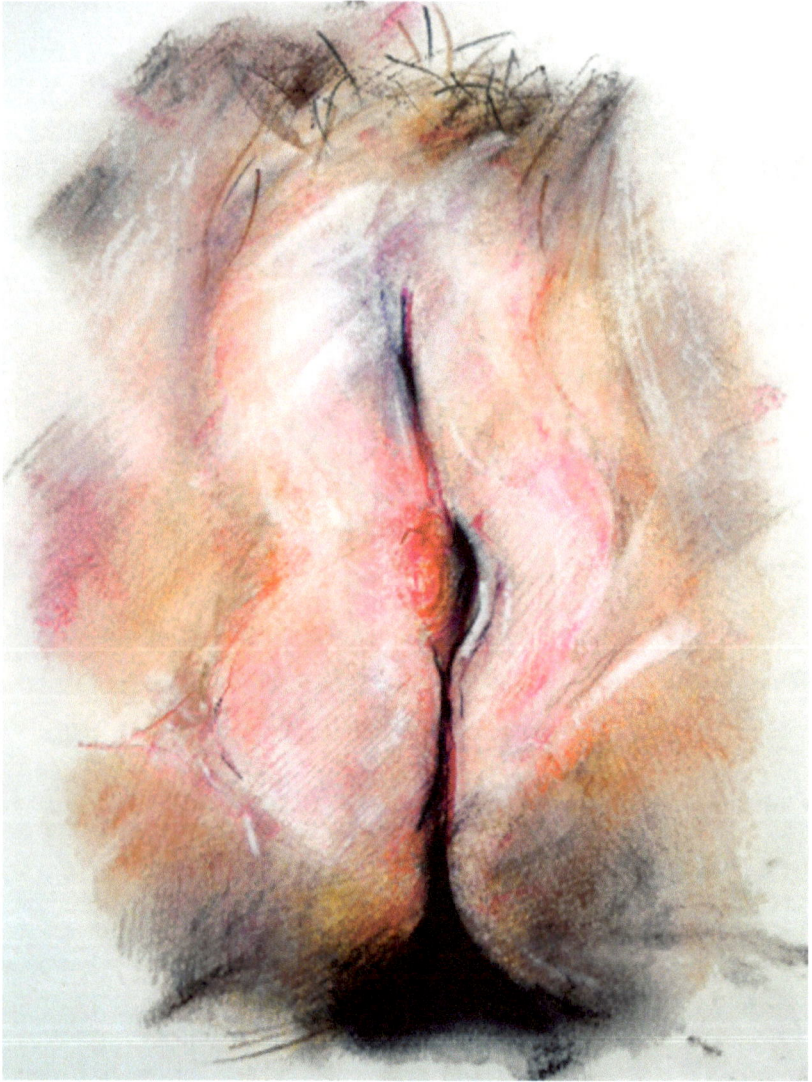

VULVA SIX WEEKS AFTER SURGERY: *coloured pencil on paper*

These three small pieces were made to illustrate an information leaflet about VIN and vulval cancer that was created as part of the *Drawing Women's Cancer* project. It was found that the majority of women involved preferred to see the drawings over photographs, which they found too objectifying, and diagrams, which they could not necessarily understand. Drawings were preferred as they 'made it look like somebody has cared'.

Reflections on 'The Cut': Part 1

It was always there, illness. I would look at Matthew and think our lives are changing because of his back and because of my cancer. I kept thinking though about the wedding, thinking what the hell were we going to do, but I was determined not to rearrange it. It was going to be something for us all to focus on.

Surgery is the standard treatment for vulval cancer, and a radical vulvectomy is the medical term used to describe an extensive surgical procedure wherein the whole of the patient's vulva, including the inner and outer lips, the deep tissue and the clitoris are removed. The patient does retain her vagina, uterus and ovaries. High morbidity (medical problems caused by the extent of the surgery) is a very real risk after such an operation, as is recurrence of the cancer, so it is best in the long run for the surgeon to take as much of the affected area away as possible. Where a 'clear margin' of healthy skin around the affected area is taken, the chances of the cancer being eradicated are markedly improved. The guiding principle is to get a margin of two centimetres, and the extensiveness of the surgery therefore depends on the size and the actual location of the tumour.

I finally met Dr D the next week. He spoke so soft and gentle. With Dr T we went through the operation again but Dr D changed a few things. Originally they were only going to take one side of the vulva away [a hemivulvectomy] but he wanted to take both sides because he said the sore patch was spreading pretty fast. They told me that I would be having a radical vulvectomy and a full reconstruction all at the same time. They said there was a small chance I would have to have a colostomy bag for the healing process but because they said percentage was tiny I wasn't too worried. Anyway, I didn't want to think about that too much. They gave me a date for my operation, the 29th June 2010. Three weeks time. They wanted to

How to cite this book chapter:
Saorsa, J. with Phillips, R. 2019. *Like Any Other Woman: The Lived Experience of Gynaecological Cancer.* Pp. 75–78. Cardiff: Cardiff University Press.
DOI: https://doi.org/10.18573/book2.n. License: CC-BY-NC-ND 4.0

give me some time to get my head around things but the really important thing I needed to know was would I be able to have children after it. They said yes. I would have to have a Caesarean section because I wouldn't be able to have a natural birth but that was OK. It was such a relief. It was the only thing I was really worried about.

Because a radical vulvectomy is such a major operation, with obvious physical and emotional repercussions, an immediate reconstruction of the vulva in the same operation, although traumatic, is often considered the best option. Naturally, surgeons always try to spare as much of the original vulva as they safely can, and where only a small amount of skin is removed it is sometimes possible to suture the remainder together. However, where larger areas are involved, skin flaps or grafts have to be made. A flap is created from the skin in an area close to the patient's vulva. Unlike a graft, which involves the surgeon taking a piece of skin from a totally different part of the body – the inner thighs, for example, or the belly – a flap is not totally disconnected from the surrounding skin. Instead it is 'rotated' onto the vulval area in order to cover the wound made by the removal of the cancer. Where such 'local flaps' can be used for vulvar reconstruction, there are definite advantages both for the surgeons and, most importantly, for the patient. Local flaps are as narrow in width as is possible, they are easily manipulable, and because they retain an attachment to the surrounding skin the blood supply to them is easier to direct and control.

I went into hospital the day before my operation because I was going to theatre first thing the next day. I know it probably sounds strange but I wasn't scared. I think it was because I didn't really know what to expect. That night lying in my hospital bed all I could think of was what if I have to have a colostomy bag. My mind was a whirlwind and I didn't really sleep tidy. First thing in the morning Matthew and my mother were by my side and I was already for theatre. Dr T and Dr D came in to discuss a few things with me. They needed to know that I fully understood what was going to happen. I knew that I had to have an epidural to keep me numb and that the operation was going to take some time. The only question I wanted to ask was, 'Will I wake up with a colostomy bag?' The percentage had somehow gone from very low to very high, so I knew then, in my heart, that I would wake up with one. Matthew and my mother gave me such a big kiss and then they were gone.

In Becky's case, the original plan was to carry out a partial vulvectomy, but the surgeons later decided, on reflection, that a full radical vulvectomy with an immediate reconstruction of the vulva would be the best approach. This inevitably increased the chances of Becky having to have a colostomy. The reconstruction would use skin flaps taken from her buttocks in what is known as a butterfly incision or, more prosaically, a modified gluteal fold V-Y advancement flap, and so, after the vulvectomy was complete, and while she was still under anaesthetic, the plastic surgeon drew the shape and dimensions of the flaps onto the skin of Becky's buttocks, on both sides, with a blue felt marker. The flaps were triangular in shape, with the base sharing the already cut edge of the vulvectomy and the apex on the line of the gluteal fold, where her buttock meets her thigh. This fold line thus described the centre of each flap. The surgeon then made incisions along the drawn lines and lifted Becky's skin, separating it from the underlying tissue and her gluteus muscle but leaving the upper corner of the flap intact, still attached by a small connecting part to the surrounding skin. This would become a 'hinge' or 'pivot point' that allowed him to pick up each flap and, with as little skin tension as possible, 'swing' it around the hinge to sew it into place, thereby creating, or rather reconstructing, Becky's vulva. Once this was done, the surgeon could close the donor sites, the areas on Becky's buttocks from which he had taken the flaps, and he did this carefully and precisely with two layers of stitching, one for the deep tissue and one for the skin.

The first surgeon had to cut to a significant depth in order to remove Becky's vulva during the radical vulvectomy, and, because of the trauma her body underwent due to the operation itself and that caused by the reconstruction, the colostomy procedure was unavoidable and was carried out at the same time. A colostomy involves one end of the colon, which is part of the bowel, being diverted to the outside of the body through an opening in the abdomen called a stoma. A plastic pouch is then placed over the stoma, and the diversion ensures that bodily waste is not passed through the rectum but is collected in the pouch. It is clearly an uncomfortable situation to have to deal with, both physically and emotionally, and, especially after such a traumatic operation, waking up with a colostomy bag was initially mortifying for Becky, for all kinds of reasons. Nevertheless, it was necessary for her healing process, and the surgeons assured her that it was temporary.

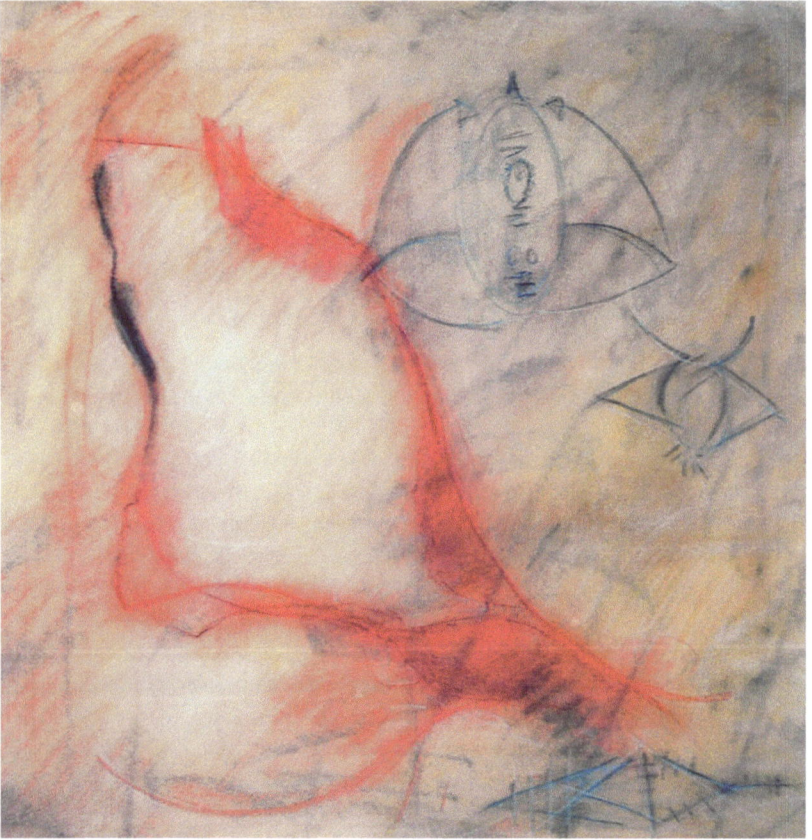

THE CUT: *chalk pastel on paper*

This drawing is my response to the surgeon's description of the nature of a radical vulvectomy followed by reconstruction, which was the operation that Becky underwent for
vulval cancer. The red lines denote the actual cuts that have to be made, and the blue
lines overlaying the 'flesh' are taken directly from the surgeon's own diagrams as she
talked me through the procedure.

I came by the horror naturally. Surgery is the one branch of medicine that is the most violent. After all, it's violent to take up a knife and cut open a person's body.

Richard Selzer

SUTURE 5: Tracey. Cervical Cancer

The procedure

Only 20 minutes ago I was talking with her as she lay in bed on the hospital ward, waiting to be called down to theatre. It was our second meeting. The first was in the clinic, last week, when she told me about her experiences since diagnosis and gave me permission to attend her operation. She looked small and vulnerable under the thin covers, but she smiled for me as I came in. It was a weak, anxious smile and I recognised the fear in her eyes, I had seen it in others before her. She seemed to appreciate the company and we had a brief conversation, talking about nothing much, the weather, what we've been up to since last we met, chatting as two people often do when there is an emotional elephant in the room.

Tracey's is a difficult story, one of disappointment and pain. When she began to notice something was wrong 'down there' she tried to ignore the physical symptoms, 'for the children'. She convinced herself it was just something minor, no need for a doctor, but she got tired of pretending that everything was OK and so, finally, she did go for help. She lives in west Wales, some distance from the nearest city, so she went to the local hospital, and to her relief they told her that there was nothing seriously wrong after all. Just abnormal cells, they said, nothing too much to worry about. But they still organised an appointment for her, here at the hospital in Cardiff, for a biopsy. She didn't understand. 'They said there was nothing wrong.' But they would give her no more information about why she was being referred, and, even though they said not to worry, she did anyway. She worried about being in the city. She worried about her two small sons at home. She worried about being alone at the hospital. She worried she might die.

It is cervical cancer, quite advanced. She is to undergo a radical hysterectomy. The whole of her uterus and the surrounding tissue, the cervix and the upper part of her vagina are to be removed. The ovaries too, probably.

How to cite this book chapter:
Saorsa, J. with Phillips, R. 2019. *Like Any Other Woman: The Lived Experience of Gynaecological Cancer.* Pp. 81–95. Cardiff: Cardiff University Press.
    DOI: https://doi.org/10.18573/book2.o. License: CC-BY-NC-ND 4.0

Reality hit hard a few weeks after the biopsy. It came suddenly, by accident, in a phone call. She is a primary school teacher and she was leading a croco-dile of children across a road into the playground. The consultant's secretary on the phone told her that she had a tumour, that she had cancer. The sec-retary assumed that she already knew, at least that she had guessed, but she didn't, she hadn't. 'It was the shock!' She can remember leaning against the playground wall and feeling as if the ground beneath her feet was giving way. She was falling, but the crocodile of children wrapped itself around her, saved her. The word, 'cancer', still makes her cry.

She has no partner and is bringing up her two young sons alone. She has not been for a smear test in years. She said, 'I haven't been active in that way, not for ages. I really thought there was no need.' And she lowered her eyes. She would not look at me as she said, 'I feel stupid now.' Now, waiting to go down to theatre, her eyes welled up as she whispered the word that makes her cry. I only nodded my head to show I understood because there were no words, just images and grief. She whispered again. 'It was the shock.'

She is asleep now, breathing gently, artificially, under the lights in theatre. They are harsh lights, but not hurtful to the eye, just very bright. They seem to illuminate even my thoughts as the huge circular structures from which they descend become acutely and disturbingly present, not just here in the room but even more powerfully in my memory. The monstrous size of them and their pitiless invasion of bodies and souls still haunt me, despite my efforts to exorcise the horror of my own experience in the weeks that followed it as I explored the depths of loss and grief through an explosion of paint on can-vas. And, for the sake of my artist's soul, I tried to find a way to let my body absolve itself of blame. I am anxious then, for Tracey, for me, for us both. This particular procedure remains very close to the emotional surface of my own consciousness, and my presence here, although willing, has psychological associations that I can neither ignore nor supplant with rational thought, so deeply are they rooted. This is a test then to the personal limit of my focus on subjective experience. Dr T knows this of me. She asked when we arranged this visit. 'Are you going to be OK with this one?' and I felt the same way I did when she asked the very first question, the one that kick-started the whole *Drawing Women's Cancer* project. She said then, 'Can you draw what it feels like to have gynaecological cancer, rather than just what it looks like?' and I only knew that I wanted to try.

Dr T is working with a colleague for this operation, and he reaches up to the light above the operating table, angling the bulbs so that they directly illuminate the inert body beneath them, clothed now in green sheeting, belly exposed. The bulbs are surrounded by protective sheaths so that he does not burn his hands, themselves tightly gloved in blue plastic. His hands are so very important.

I stand back as they begin to push gauze wadding into Tracey's vagina. This is the packing: they cannot have the vagina move during the operation, and the packing pushes it up towards the uterus, making the whole area more accessible for the surgeon. In the process however it feels as if Tracey, the patient, has to become an object, no longer a woman, a primary school teacher, a mother. I ask about the pile of gauze left on the floor between Dr T's feet. She answers in a whisper, almost conspiratorial. 'It's to protect from the excess. I pushed too hard once. I was in training and I was so scared of the consultant… we noticed that there was a lot of blood just dripping out onto the floor'. She is smiling as she recounts this tale, and I suspect, I hope, that it is a little overblown, but even so the pushing and the packing seem endless.

Dr T finally finishes the preliminaries and goes to a side room to attend to the paperwork. Her colleague is left to make the first cut. It is firm and certain, vertical, from the navel to the pubic bone. He draws the diatherm (a type of electrical 'scalpel') slowly, painfully, through the skin of the belly, which trembles around the small part of it that is taut and stretched between his fingers. 'A cut needs tension.' I am surprised that he uses a diatherm for this initial cut, deep and long as it has to be, so I ask. 'Yes,' he replies with confidence. He is more than willing to explain the process to me, and he demonstrates his professionalism in the way that, as he talks, his eyes never leave the cut. 'It's the way we do it now.' There is a slight pause as he draws the diatherm through a difficult section. 'But some surgeons do still use a scalpel.'

The edges of the cut sizzle and blacken as he works, simultaneously cutting and cauterising the flesh. Smoke and the acrid smell of burnt flesh arise from the wound that becomes bigger, deeper as he cuts, confidently, deftly, down through layers of yellow fat. As the belly opens, my artist's eye focuses on how the colours that move through the wound, from the skin, through the fat and the connective tissue to the fleshy muscle, are aesthetically so beautiful in harmonious juxtaposition. First the hues of red: crimson, napthol and the brightest perylene intermingling with tiny glimpses of green and blue, the colours of the shadows on the flesh. And then on through the spectrum of yellow, from the deepest cadmium to the palest, prettiest lemon, the colours of the daffodils that are blooming outside, flowers that bear so much significance here in Wales. *Cenhinen* (ken-HIN-en) means 'leek' in Welsh, while *cenhinen bedr* (ken-HIN-en BED-er) means daffodil, or St Peter's leek. Over the length of history the two became confused until the daffodil was finally adopted as a second national emblem of Wales. The *cenhinen bedr* then are blooming today, even as the wound is opened and the fat gives way, melting under the surgeon's hand.

Watching, in awe, I think of *Chroma*, the book by Derek Jarman (2000), painter and filmmaker, in which he extends Melville's view that we learn colour while not necessarily understanding it. But it is understanding that I am seeking here, in subjective form, and in the wound as I watch it open, the red of the initial cut becomes Jarman's 'moment in time … quickly spent. An explosion of intensity.' Further on, as the diatherm moves down through the soft tissue, the intensity of the red 'burns itself. Disappears like fiery sparks into the gathering shadow.' Jarman imagined four stages distinguishable in alchemy: the blackening of 'melanosis', the whitening of 'leucosis', the yellowing of 'xanthosis' and the reddening of 'iosis'. For me, as I gaze into human depths, they all appear as the diatherm cuts beyond borders, through bloody barriers, deeper and deeper into the body, opening it up and invading its private, once autonomous spaces. I feel the sting. And Jarman says, 'Painters use red like spice.'

Dr T returns, bringing even more paper wadding to mop up the excess. 'Excess: an amount of something that is more than necessary, permitted, or desirable' (Oxford English Dictionary). Excess is here, then, even beyond the metastasising cancer that in itself is excess to normal cell structure. Excess indeed, excess that needs to be curtailed, constrained, cut out... extirpated.

Standing on a stool to get a better view, I watch as the surgeon cuts deeper into the now-exposed muscle. The rectus abdominis yields to the unrelenting diatherm and gives access to the peritoneum and the abdominal cavity. There it is, the uterus, itself now destined to become 'excess'. Dr T delves into the open abdomen and lifts it out, cradling it in her hand. 'Look,' she says as she gently offers it up. 'And here.' She points into the void. 'Here the ovaries.'

Fat, organs, tissue, all that was inside is now outside, spilling over the edges of the gaping wound, colours mingling at all levels of the warm scale as the surgeons work with cold concentration. I am shocked. No, not shocked, more bemused as I witness what appears as a mess, a fluid jumble of organs that belies the naïve impression, that I now realise I have always held, that inside we are all very orderly and self-contained. Art takes precedence over science here as the boundary between order and disorder becomes confused. I think of the ouroboros symbol that I carry tattooed on my shoulder, a symbol of the eternal unity of all things, the cycle of birth and death and the encircling of chaos with order, but either way the art–science relationship is here emphatically demonstrated through an ideal of structure, the structure of the human body, which becomes simultaneous with function through an overall concept of process. I allow myself to disappear (escape?) into a corner of philosophy where a conversation I once had with Gilles Deleuze and Paul Ricoeur still matters, but I must return; I must bear witness to what is happening in front of me.

Both surgeons together push Tracey's visceral organs around with their hands, bullying them into compliance as they push them up towards the diaphragm, the dome-shaped muscular partition that mercifully seals off the chest cavity. They need to isolate the uterus, but the body is tenacious, the organs persistently spilling back out of the wound as if defending, even nurturing the one among them that is the object of attention. Yet more gauze wadding is forced into the body to hold back the tide, to create defensive embankments that extend upwards to the ribcage and down towards the pelvis. Finally, with his arm up to the elbow inside the passive form, like Canute on the shore, the surgeon pushes and shoves with a physical force that is continuously ineffectual but promises a painful recovery.

I am stunned by the seeming violence of it all, the brutality, the deeply and intensely visceral reality of the scene before me. The edges of the wound are pulled wider open with clamps that grasp the bloodied flesh and become bloodied in their turn. Now the diatherm, held lightly first in one surgeon's hand, then in the other's, probes and cuts on respective sides of the pelvic cavity, an empty space that they have created now devoid of organs and 'excess' save the hapless uterus, the one which is soon to become the 'other'. It sits isolated, bounded by smooth, slippery walls of Tracey's abdominal cavity that shine and appear translucent yet simultaneously opaque. It looks so small, so vulnerable under the threat of the diatherm, and the ovaries, white and tiny, are hiding, sheltering, in the darkness of the void.

Witnessing the procedure is salutary in terms of my understanding. The pushing, the shoving, the manipulation of the body structures and organs, the bloodied tools that are first discarded, then retrieved, then put into service to cut, to staple, to open and to close, all this is played out in front of me in sanguine ritual. The same blood pools in the crevices of the body and on the floor at the surgeons' feet. Small bits of the flesh that it once made red are thrown up onto the green sheet, or down into the pools. This is not clean, not clinical. This is raw, visceral, almost primeval. It feels... it *feels*. This is the unadulterated, non-sugar-coated authenticity of surgery. The cutting, the slicing, the pushing and the pulling, the packing, the mopping up... and it is all the raw bloodiness of real flesh, real wounds. It is nature, rent and protesting. The body, once a closed space of quietude and privacy, is now wide open, stretched, clamped and 'mined' for the tumours that threaten its very existence as they turn the acting Self (that part of being human which here, in this theatre, on this table, is absent) into Sontag's 'Non-Self'. I draw nearer to see as best I can while being careful to avoid any contact with the green sheet that protects the human being, Tracey, who has become subject to (or is it perhaps object to?) this therapeutic violation. Standing close beside the surgeon, I have a clear view of how she works, now with force, now with gentleness, but always with dominance. The body submits. Once the surface and the underlying defences have been breached there is little to resist the relentless subjugation of its autonomy. In stark contrast to the violence being perpetrated, Tracey's chest is rising and falling gently, passively. Its normality and regularity, at least in this respect, is confirmed by the anaesthetist, who lays his hand protectively on her shoulder as he watches the fluctuations of his parallel, and multicoloured, digital lines.

Two hours in and the surgeons begin to work more slowly. Brutality is replaced in the details by delicacy and the sensitivity that must dictate the smallest and most intimate of incisions. The cancer may not have settled only in the cervix; there may be subsidiaries, and so they need to explore, to single out the pelvic lymph nodes, the arteries, the nerves. Like Selzer's (1996) predators on the prowl, the surgeons, the hunters, move quietly, deliberately, stalking the prey, the obscure lumps of flesh that have become firm to the touch and are thus differentiated from the soft masses within which they are concealed. The main tumour will be taken coldly and cleanly with the uterus, an eradication of the very taproot of the cancer's existence, but the morbid and innately malignant potentiality may still lie in the lymph nodes that now become vulnerable, unprotected by innocent flesh as the surgeons delve with life-preserving precision into the depths of the body, first one side then the other, moving slowly. They are suspicious. They search carefully, steadily and without pity, isolating, feeling, cutting, debating and moving on, constantly aware of how far they can to go before breaching a physical boundary impossible to cross with any hope of returning. They take various samples, all of which 'feel' benign, and then, suddenly, there it is. A tiny lump of bloody flesh is dropped into a plastic vial and a phone call is made. This is a sample they suspect but cannot be sure of. They need to do a frozen section, and the operation has to be delayed while they await the result of the analysis because, they tell me, 'If it's positive, there's no point in going on'. I feel suddenly very cold, although it is warm in the theatre. They switch off the lights.

Four hours in and we are still waiting for the lab results. One of the surgeons goes to perform another operation, the next patient on her list, while her first lies, covered in green cloth, but with the wound open, exposed, and packed with the ubiquitous gauze wadding. I have to leave – life draws me back to a world outside the theatre – but I feel I am living in some kind of parallel reality until I receive a text later in the evening from the surgeon.

Tracey was under anaesthetic for a total of eight hours. The sample was negative and the surgeons completed the hysterectomy. They left one ovary.

Radiotherapy

There is only a bare minimum of recovery time after the hysterectomy before Tracey has to begin radiotherapy treatment. The surgery went well but she has to undergo a course of radiotherapy followed by one week of brachytherapy to ensure that all the cancer has been eradicated. The number of sessions, one every weekday for five weeks then one every day for one week, comes as a surprise to her. 'It's so long a time,' she says with dismay, although her doctor has told her that it is the standard dosage.

> **Radiotherapy** is a treatment where radiation is used to kill cancer cells. There are many different ways you can have radiotherapy, but they all work in a similar way. They damage cancer cells and stop them from growing or spreading in the body. Radiotherapy is generally considered the most effective cancer treatment after surgery, but how well it works varies from person to person. (NHS website)
>
> **Brachytherapy** uses radioactive implants such as seeds, pellets, wires or plates that are put near or inside the tumour. A high dose of radiation is

given to the tumour, but nearby healthy areas get much less. In the case of cervical cancer, hollow tubes are placed into the vagina. One end of each tube sits inside the vagina or womb. The other end sits outside the body between the patient's legs. The ends of the tubes outside the body are connected to a treatment machine. The machine sends a radioactive pellet into each tube. It keeps the pellets in the tubes in the vagina or womb to give the treatment. When the treatment has finished the pellets return to the machine. (Macmillan Cancer Support website)

The hospital is some 40 minutes' drive from her home. As there is nobody able to come with her on a regular basis, or to look after her young sons, she has to come alone and organise her appointments for during school hours so that she can get back to collect them. She says that the staff have been very obliging and she assures me that she will be fine. A friend might come with her for the first session, and maybe for a couple of times after that, but I definitely have an uneasy sense of... What? Responsibility? No, not that. But what then? I don't know for sure but I tell myself that it doesn't matter as I offer to meet her myself at the hospital for at least some of her visits. I am thinking of how I might feel in her situation... Is that even possible? Can I, with any integrity, imagine what she might feel? But she accepts my offer readily and seems almost excited by the idea of my continuing to write about her ongoing experiences. I realise then that our relationship is set to take a new turn around the complex issue of the duality of purpose that has always been a driving force behind the *Drawing Women's Cancer* project as a whole. The realisation turns into questions that I ask myself as I arrive at the clinic on the second day of her treatment. Why am I here? Why am I doing this? And the answers come with less assurance than I would like. To support her, of course; she would be alone in this otherwise, but I am also here to continue the aims of the project, to try to express the experience of illness more profoundly through word and image by following through and witnessing her continuing treatment. I am not fully convinced. Again. What then is our new relationship?

This situation, like many others during the project, forces me to fully appreciate that the idea of academic research and the questions of methodology and rationale that served to validate the project in the beginning have become, if not obsolete, at least very inadequate in terms of the work that I am doing. Ethical considerations are important, of course, but they are tacit, and none of the women I have worked with had much interest in the forms I have had to ask them to sign as confirmation of their consent to be involved. So, where the researcher/subject relationship is far too abject a concept to represent what is really going on here, and where such human separateness is only a tenuous ideal anyway within the intimacy and humanity of shared experience, in the work that I am doing and the relationships I am making, surely common decency, even at the most basic level, along with the shared sense of humanity and respect for one another easily silences the intones of any form of contrived clinical detachment. Such formality can then, at least sometimes, be legitimately left to the medics.

For Tracey and I, therefore, our relationship begins to explore a rich geology of experience wherein many layers of narrative become deposits that sometimes run parallel and sometimes collide. Even where one layer may obscure another in the tortuous agony of a sedimentary fold, it constantly forms and reforms the bedrock under a landscape of unadulterated humanity that lies between us. Of course I want to be supportive in a difficult time, but in my being so I know that we will talk and laugh together, swap stories of life and of experience in general, and, during the process, I will, at times, be conscious of being very open and of perhaps leaving myself almost as vulnerable as she is. But we are two human beings, one in pain, the other empathetic. Both of us sharing the responsibility and contributing to the narrative about our separate experiences of the other, unwelcome character in the plot – her cancer. This is the power of narrative to express humanity, which is derived from and, above all, is characterised by mutual subjectivity.

We had agreed to meet in the reception, and as I arrive, early, I receive a text from her telling me she is on her way. The clinic is surprisingly crowded, and I feel oddly conspicuous so I resort to checking emails on my phone, hoping that such a ubiquitous act might help me feel less out of place. When Tracey arrives I notice that she looks surprisingly well considering what she has already been through, and then I wonder exactly what I had really been expecting. After a brief 'hello' we go through to the radiotherapy waiting area, where it is much quieter than in the reception, and find two seats close to the window. She begins to tell me about her first visit here, the previous day, and says that, although she is pleasantly surprised that the individual session itself is quite painless and takes only around 15 minutes, at the same time she is disappointed that the treatment as a whole will take so long to complete. She tells me how she hopes the brachytherapy, which will be done at another hospital even further away from her home, will follow on immediately because she is worried about not finishing in time for the school holidays.

As yet she has not heard about appointment dates for the brachytherapy, but she shows me the schedule for her radiotherapy sessions, and we agree on the dates that I will be able to be with her here. I curse inwardly because my next week is full of studio commitments and I am still insecure enough about what I am doing to worry about whether she thinks I don't care. But she seems happy for anything that I can do, and so we make our plans. Tracey knows that it takes me an hour or so to get to the clinic, and she says that she worries about me 'wasting my time'. She is looking for reassurance and I offer it without question.

Her appointment time passes and we are still waiting so she starts to tell me about her meeting with a doctor the day before. She says that the doctor was 'a bit abrupt and not very understanding' as she wrote out a prescription for a medication for diarrhoea. It is obvious then what side effects she might expect from the radiotherapy, and we cheerfully discuss the practicalities of this for her drive home. She laughs easily, but her smile belies the confusion and the worry she is feeling, the difficulties she has faced in the short time between the operation and the start of this treatment and the fact that now, despite having struggled to feel stronger and normal again, she now feels 'like a patient again'. I see... no, I *feel* the emotion she is keeping down, the tears just beneath the surface. Suddenly her name is called and with a rueful smile she is gone.

I look around the waiting room from my vantage point by the window. It is clean and functional, with high-backed chairs around the walls and rows of smaller chairs in the centre, all upholstered in a dark blue material that is, in some places, becoming slightly worn. Colourful prints of flowers and nondescript landscapes hang listlessly on the walls, and beside my chair there is a wire rack holding magazines about celebrity lifestyles, gardening tips and DIY, along with information leaflets about various types of cancer. More of the chairs are now occupied as people arrive for their appointments. Some are alone, while others sit with companions, carers, husbands, wives. With the exception of some obvious cases, it is difficult to determine who are patients and who are not, but everybody is waiting for names to be called by nurses who appear and disappear with surprising regularity. Some people are chatting, even laughing, some are reading newspapers or peering at their phones. Some seem lost in their own unique and individual reverie, but overall there is an almost tangible air of restrained emotion degenerating into resignation. Most look tired, careworn, and I feel a very real and communal sense of loss that simply cannot be contained in the small room.

A couple enter. I guess that they are middle-aged, although they both look much older. She is physically tiny, with a grey pallor punctuated by darkened shadows under her eyes and cheekbones. She is huddled in a wheelchair, her arms hanging limply, almost unnaturally, from her thin shoulders that protrude sharply from under a thick shawl that is loosely wrapped around her frail body. Like a shroud, I think to myself. He is tall and, like her, painfully thin. His face is drawn and his expression a mixture of exhausted compassion and frustration. Pausing at the entrance of the waiting area, he leans over her, saying something to her in a low whisper, and in reply she slowly raises a skeletal hand and points to the window. He nods, straightens up and obediently pushes her towards where I am sitting. Parking her wheelchair in the aisle, next to the row of chairs directly opposite me, he bends to put on the brake before taking a seat beside her. I smile politely at them both, and he responds reluctantly with a quick nod. I feel a little self-conscious, not knowing quite what to do, but then she gifts me with a smile so wide and so full of warmth that I feel honoured to be in the company of someone who is clearly suffering but who can still find the courage to be so generous, even to a complete stranger.

Only a few minutes pass before a nurse approaches the couple. She looks anxious, harassed. The man gets quickly to his feet, expectant, but the news is that there is no bed available and they will have to wait while she, the nurse, tries to 'sort something out'. The man seems to shrink, to close in on himself. He asks how long they will have to wait but receives no positive answer, and as his frustration begins to take form, his charge shifts a little in her chair. She reaches out to him in an obvious effort to calm the situation as the nurse stammers an apology and hurries away. The couple seem to teeter on the edge of an argument, but it is an unrealised threat. His fractious responses to her soothing tones seem to come less from anger than from a sense of impotence, and they belie the love and care that, though obviously tested to the limit, still remain firm and clearly expressed in the way his hand now clasps hers, held in frail tension in her lap. I feel strangely weak, depleted. It is as if the whole range of emotions is being played out just a few feet from me and all I can do is witness it.

Tracey returns from her treatment and smiles as she sees me hurriedly putting away my notebook. I don't know why I feel so guilty about it; after all, she knows full well that I am writing all this down. We go to the hospital café, where we drink tea and eat cake, and we laugh; there is always laughter. We are sitting by the window and the summer sun is burning with such force through the glass that it is almost too hot to bear, but the conversation rides a roller-coaster through many levels and many emotions as I feel the sweat begin to run down my back. We are getting to know each other better. We are talking about the project and about my drawing, my writing. She has already read the narrative about her operation and has no objections to it being published: she wants the story told. There will eventually be a book. I promise her. She says, 'Put this in the book.'

Radiotherapy day 11

I arrive early as usual so I ask for a cup of tea at the WRVS café while I wait. But I have only a £10 note to pay for a mug of tea that costs just 60 pence and I feel awkward as the assistant studiously counts out my change, all in small coin. When Tracey arrives we walk through to the waiting room and she tells me about the intense back pain she has experienced over the past week. It's been a 'bad week'. She looks tired, worn down. Suddenly she spots a friend across the room, a woman she has met before here on a day I was unable to come. With a brief, unnecessary apology she goes over, and as they talk, clearly 'swapping notes', the two women become animated, each visibly shedding the attitude of vulnerable patient and replacing it with an energy born of shared experience. From across the room it seems a very intimate exchange, almost conspiratorial, and I am happy for her as I know that a friend who is going through a similar thing can surely offer better emotional support than I can. But Friend's husband looks uncomfortable. Perhaps he is feeling the anxiety of an exile, cast out even if only temporarily from a world that even to enter in the first place must have taken so very much from him. Friend has breast cancer.

Tracey looks happier now. As she crosses the room again to sit beside me she is smiling again and I feel her spirit lifting. I have claimed our usual two seats by the window, and as the sun begins to shine through the glass she tells me that she now has her dates for the brachytherapy treatment and it is a relief to know that it will run straight after the radiotherapy. She needs to go for five sessions and there are only two that clash with when the boys will be on their school holiday. It's not going to be as awkward then as she had feared, at least in practical terms.

Her name is called.

As I am waiting for her and making some notes, another woman who had been sitting across from me returns from her own treatment. I notice that she looks brighter than when she went in. Relief maybe? Her husband, who has been sitting quietly alone with his thoughts while she's been gone, just looks hurt, deeply, as if he has been so for a long time. The woman busies herself with her bag, her scarf, her thick coat, and it strikes me that the oddness of this, given the exceptionally warm weather we are having, is poignant. When she is ready they prepare to leave and as they go she gives me a friendly nod. The whole scenario seems strangely normal, but I remind myself that for them this has probably become normality. After all, they have to do it every day.

Friend also returns from her treatment and, although her husband clearly wants to leave immediately, she starts up a conversation with another waiting couple. I cannot, and indeed do not want to, hear the actual words, but the body language says it all. The conversation animates the two women just as I saw it do between Friend and Tracey. It is clear that Friend is trying earnestly to reassure the other woman. She is lifting up her arm and pointing to where I imagine her own tumour had once been. The other woman reciprocates, and I have a twinge of guilt about having the feeling that I am witnessing a bizarre form of illness one-upmanship! In a few moments, less than 15 this time, Tracey returns. She is suddenly emotional, the tears she's been keeping down are finally surfacing and they cause her voice to break. 'Everything is catching up with me. I feel so out of control. I'm feeling really ill now where I felt strong and well just before this treatment started.' She tells me that she worries that the people she is seeing here are 'far worse off' than her and that 'I've had it easy really'. I only listen, letting her talk, because I sense that it would not be of much help to her just at this moment if I tried to persuade her otherwise, however true it might be. I have to simply give her the space to tell me how she feels; she gets little opportunity to do that after all. But Friend is still here and she comes over, clearly seeing another opportunity to reassure. Tracey seems happy she is there but they actually say nothing to each other; they only hug for a long time. Afterwards, as Tracey and I get ready to leave, Friend catches my eye and gives me a knowing look.

As this is an appointment where the doctor has to review Tracey's treatment and her progress we have to go through to the next clinic and begin another wait. In fact, we have to wait for some time, and so, in an effort to take her mind off her own reality, I talk a lot about my week past and, perhaps bizarrely, about how I tend my ever-expanding collection of cacti! There is laughter and she is smiling again. The distraction works, even if only for a while.

After she has seen the doctor she has to go to the pharmacy to collect her prescription, and so once again we have to wait. The pharmacy reception is a small, claustrophobic room with no windows and a strange pervasive smell that neither of us can recognise and neither of us really wants to. The sun is strong again today, and this cell of a room is becoming unbearably hot. To make things worse, there is no way to keep the automatic entrance door open to let in any air. Even the door itself is an instrument of torture in that it screeches in unoiled agony every time someone enters or leaves. The awful sound pierces through every fibre of my being and sets my teeth on edge. We marvel at the fact that we have to wait nearly 30 minutes for a small packet that the nurse simply takes off the shelf, especially as the packet itself was remarkably already similar to the packet in her bag that she bought at Boots just yesterday. Even though here she gets it for free, we debate on whether the wait is actually worth the small saving she's made.

Eventually we are released, as though from the eighth circle of hell, and we head for the café as before. This time we choose a table further inside as the sun is still beating relentlessly through the window in the corner and we've had enough of heat. Over tea and Chelsea buns we talk a lot about her life and her relationships, but mostly about her two small boys. She loves them deeply, unreservedly, and with all her heart and soul.

Radiotherapy day 16

Tracey again seems worn down and tired when we meet in the waiting room. She tells me that the unrelenting back pain is now combined with a constant sensation of bloating. She has not been able to eat much. She says that the radiotherapy staff told her last week that she had lost weight, and although she is pleased about this on one level, there are mixed emotions.

I'm worried that I am late as she is here before me, but she was told the previous day apparently that she to come an hour earlier for her appointment so that she could see the doctor for yet another review. But she's still waiting. I sit down and we giggle together as she explains her 'bladder issues' and the lengths she has to go to in order to makes sure she is always within reach of a toilet. She seems to cheer up a little as we talk and she tells me how she feels so embarrassed when her mother brings her remedies for diarrhoea that have been suggested by well-meaning friends. 'Flat coke and marshmallows! Put that in the book!' Finally her name is called but it isn't to see the doctor; it is for her regular radiotherapy session. With a heavy sigh and a 'why did I bother to get here early?' look on her face, she follows the nurse into the treatment room.

The waiting room is busy today. Unusually there are lots of men here, some alone, some waiting with partners or wives, mothers or friends, but there is also one woman sitting alone, apart from everyone else. She is very thin, almost skeletal, and dressed in a hospital gown over flower-patterned pyjamas. Her small feet are pushed into slippers that are obviously not big enough, even for her, and are consequently beaten down at the heels where she has walked on them. She is wearing a red woollen beanie that I assume is intended to disguise the baldness that comes as an unwelcome accomplice to chemotherapy, and she has a scarf wrapped tightly around her neck. She is clearly uncomfortable, alone in the waiting room, and seems to be very self-conscious. Her eyes under naked brows dart around the room as she turns her hands in her lap, her fingers whitening at the knuckles. I feel slightly guilty as I cast equally furtive glances in her direction, but from my artist's point of view the whole manner of her being becomes a catalyst for so many images and I can't help myself. After a few moments, however, another woman enters from the far side of the room. She is also alone and she walks very slowly and carefully towards the nearest chair. When she reaches it she seems to simply let herself fall, with no real control over her movements, and once seated she grips the arms of the chair very tightly. Like the other woman she is also wearing a hospital gown and a woolly beanie, blue this time. A nurse comes over to her and says something very quietly. Then she briefly lays her hand on the woman's shoulder. As the nurse hurries away again the woman bows her head and buries her face in her hands. More nurses come in and out calling names that are sometimes answered, sometimes not. The woman in the blue beanie just sinks lower into her chair.

Sitting opposite me there is a young man who is tapping the screen of his iPhone. I assume he is waiting for someone as he doesn't project any sense of the weariness or resignation that I have often seen accompany illness; in fact he positively radiates resilient health. For this he is a perfect example, in Sontag's terms, of a citizen of the 'Kingdom of the Well', and, while he is perhaps unaware, in his own experience, of any place like a 'Kingdom of the Sick', he seems to remain also unaware of his very powerful presence in this room that is full of sick people. I am thinking about this as I watch his thumbs flick noiselessly and incredibly quickly over the small screen, and I begin to feel very conscious of the room as itself a very powerful and emotive transitory space between two separate ways of being. In recent months I have noticed an ever-enthusiastic proclivity, especially in the arts, towards the concept of liminality, the quality of ambiguity or disorientation, the unfamiliar space that lies 'in-between' familiarity. The experience of this room, indeed of the situation as a whole, is definitely of a liminal space both in time and in emotion, but, I think, it is too 'real', too resonant of the fundamental human condition to ever fit easily into any esoteric or conceptual fad.

I am deep in thought and, as usual, making copious notes as Tracey returns from her treatment. She smiles, as she always does when she catches me scribbling. There are no tears this time, simply frustration because they have told her that the doctor cannot see her now till 1.30. Just over an hour, then, to wait. We agree that it might be best to stay around rather than go to the café and risk missing her appointment, so we get tea from the WRVS and find a quiet corner. We talk about the normal things, the weather, holidays, the coast in Wales and of course about her boys. Her sense of humour at least has remained healthy throughout all this, and we laugh a lot as we talk about anything, anything, that is, except cancer. She says she is tired of talking about her illness, tired of feeling a victim, so I tell her about how I have heard about a beach in Ceredigion where there is a submerged forest of prehistoric tree stumps. She says she always loves the way I come up with random subjects, and as the story rapidly takes on hilarious proportions I worry that perhaps our laughter might seem irreverent in this environ. But it always helps.

Radiotherapy day 21

This time she looks bad. The worst in fact that she has looked since her treatment began. The 'bladder issues' continue. 'It's like really bad cystitis now,' she says. 'And so painful too. This treatment is making me feel worse than I've ever felt.' After her session we go as usual to the café, and in the middle of the habitual chat about life in general she suddenly wants to talk about her operation. She wants to know what it felt like for me to watch it happen and she wants to talk about the difference between a hysterectomy and a 'radical' hysterectomy. She says she is confused about why they left one ovary. Maybe she wants to talk about this because it is my last day with her here; indeed, it is the last day of her radiotherapy sessions in total and in two days' time she will begin her brachytherapy at another clinic in Cardiff.

I try to explain the difference between a general procedure and a radical one, although I am wondering as I am doing so whether this isn't something that the medics should have gone through with her and made sure she understood. As for the remaining ovary, I have to admit that I am as much in the dark perhaps as she is, although I could make the assumption that as the ovary was not affected by the cancer they decided to leave it intact, however 'redundant' it may have become. Tracey thinks about this for a while and if only from the expression on her face I can feel the effort it is taking her to come to terms with things as they are. It seems to me that she hasn't fully faced up to the reality of what has happened to her, although I am reluctant to say so and risk opening doors that I'm in no position to help close. Acceptance of violation, even when it is done with the best intentions and in order to save her life, is hard, and on many levels I know only too well what she is going through. But I cannot pursue this. I am experienced in counselling, experienced enough to know that, but this is not a counselling situation. This is my last day with her and the onus is on me to keep her, and myself, safe, to bring some sort of closure rather than begin something more. So there is a silence between us, but it is not uncomfortable, and after a few moments she looks up at me and says, with the dry humour that I have come to really appreciate in her, 'Well, the ovary's nuked now anyway, nuked well and truly!' Just for a second I wondered whether to laugh or cry. Then we laugh, as we always do.

The conversation turns to 'what next', and I decide to ask how she feels about the idea of 'survivorship'. I already know that I am tiptoeing on dangerous ground here but it is something I feel I need to raise, if only for the sake of knowing that this part of our relationship at least is coming to a natural end. Her smile disappears and she says she doesn't want to think about what she is going through in those terms at all. She becomes animated, indignant. 'Do you know, I visited Maggie's Cancer Centre the other day and it was definitely not a good experience. I felt like a victim; it was all just too much in your face.' I know now that I am in the company of a woman who is very much not a victim, and I tell her so with utter conviction.

As we part, Tracey catches my arm. 'So this is the last time,' she says, handing me a parcel wrapped in paper with a paisley pattern. 'This is for you, to say thank you. Thank you for everything.' It is a notebook with daffodil-yellow covers and spiral bound. I thank her, hug her, and leave. I hope she knows how much the gift means to me. On the walk back to the car I weep.

Postscript

Tracey and I have met twice since that last day in the radiotherapy clinic. The first time we walked together along a sandy beach on the Welsh coast. We walked and talked about how she was coping in the aftermath while her sons hunted for fossils in the rocks below the layered cliffs. The second time we met she visited me in my studio. She brought me daffodils. She is cancer free and the *cenhinen bedr* burst from the ground, every spring, in yellow celebration.

Becky. Return Visit: Part 5

In theatre it's always cold! I was freezing and I had loads of doctors around me, someone was putting needles into my arm and another doctor was putting the needle into my back. I'm not going to lie, it did hurt, but there and then the doctor explained to me the epidural needle had gone in too far so when I woke up after the operation I would have to go to intensive care so they could keep an eye on me. Later on, in the recovery room I pulled the oxygen mask of my face and I asked the nurse 'Have I got a colostomy bag?' She said, 'Yes'. I was really upset about that but then I started to vomit and I felt so very tired. After an hour they moved me from recovery to intensive care where Matthew and my parents were waiting for me. They all looked wore out and they told me how long I had been gone. In total it was eleven and a half hours and they'd felt like they were going crazy having to wait all that time and then finding out I had to be taken to intensive care. I had tubes coming out of everywhere and the doctor who done the epidural wanted me to drink as much caffeine as possible because he said caffeine would stop the headaches that were the after effects of the epidural going wrong.

An accidental dural puncture (ADP) is not an uncommon complication during placement of an epidural catheter for anaesthesia and analgesia. The dura mater is one of the membranes that surround the brain and spinal cord and if it is punctured or torn in any way the patient almost inevitably suffers, among other things, a severe headache, which in medical terms is defined as a post-dural puncture headache, or PDPH.

I spent two days in intensive care before returning to the ward, but by the third day I was feeling so ill I couldn't keep anything down, not even water. Something was wrong so the ward sister asked for the doctor who done my epidural to come and see me. I have never felt so ill. I thought I was dying.

How to cite this book chapter:
Saorsa, J. with Phillips, R. 2019. *Like Any Other Woman: The Lived Experience of Gynaecological Cancer.* Pp. 97–98. Cardiff: Cardiff University Press.
DOI: https://doi.org/10.18573/book2.p. License: CC-BY-NC-ND 4.0

I was only twenty-four and I looked like a frail old woman. When the doctor saw me he knew straight away that the epidural had leaked into me.

Cerebrospinal fluid is the clear fluid that surrounds, cushions and protects both the brain and spinal cord. In an ADP, the hole or tear created can allow a leakage of this fluid into the body and this causes many problems, including an increased risk of meningitis. Although some leakages can heal of their own accord, more severe cases need to be treated.

Something needed to be done right away so they took me back to theatre to do a blood patch where they took blood from my wrist and put it into my back.

An epidural blood patch, or EBP, is a surgical procedure that uses the patient's own blood, taken from elsewhere in the body, to close a hole or tear in the dura mater of the spinal cord, where the cause has been an ADP. A blood patch is usually a very efficient way to relieve post-dural puncture headaches.

The headaches lifted almost immediately and suddenly I was feeling a lot better. I had to stay in bed for five more days and then I was allowed to get up and sit in the chair. It was time then for me to do battle with my colostomy bag. At first it was real hard for me to accept it. The nurses were teaching me how to empty my bag and how to change it and I got real upset over it, I just didn't want to do it, but I knew I had to because if I didn't I wouldn't be allowed home. That made me determined to get over what I was feeling and manage it.

Dr T came to see how I was doing. I had a lot of stitches in my bum area because of the reconstruction and she explained to me that she had had to cut a bit deeper than she expected. But the operation was a success. Good news! A few days before I was due to come home I wanted to have a look down below to see what it looked like. I was amazed by what they'd done, it was so neat. I really didn't expect the reconstruction to look like that at all. I thought they'd done a brilliant job.

Although Becky's first operation was successful in that it destroyed the cancer, it was described as radical for good reason. The surgery to remove her vulva and then to reconstruct it left her with physical scars, which will heal in time, and emotional wounds, which are much slower to close, if indeed they ever will. Healing has become an extended and continually problematic process.

Reflections on 'The Cut': Part 2

In all of my conversations with Becky she was never very forthcoming about the details of her diagnosis, other than it was for vulval cancer, and I realised at the time that, for her, the actual nature of the disease was far less important than recovering from it, and from its consequences, which, although she couldn't have known at the time, were to be far-reaching. Added to this, her faith in the medical team who were dealing with her case, and indeed in the medical profession and in our NHS in general, was without doubt unshakeable. But this was to change: her faith was set to waver, her trust betrayed, but nobody knew that then and, given the shocking news, Becky suddenly had no thoughts for the future. At that time, in her present, what she had was a cancer diagnosis, and what she needed was the strength to survive it.

It is a traumatic assault, in and on every sense. Even if it was half expected, a cancer diagnosis takes our normality, as we understand it, and violently knocks it out of kilter. In good health, all of the assumptions and expectations of a future, all of the 'taken-for-grantedness' and the 'it'll-never-happen-to-me-ness' can protect us like a comfortable security blanket, but a cancer diagnosis can tear the blanket aside and leave us naked to the elements, wounded and vulnerable, standing on the frontier between Sontag's 'Kingdom of the Well' and 'Kingdom of the Sick' (Sontag 1990). Just as we are all individuals, we all react in different ways to such an experience, and Becky's way was to give over her trust and her body to the professionals, simply, obediently following their lead without needing to ask many questions. Her strength of mind is clear for all to see in the way in which she did so without complaint, but that was then. Fortunately, for me now, because details are important in order for me to understand her experiences as closely as I can and because I do ask questions, she is happy when I ask to share what few medical notes that she has. Our text conversation about my request is brief, her answer enlightening.

How to cite this book chapter:
Saorsa, J. with Phillips, R. 2019. *Like Any Other Woman: The Lived Experience of Gynaecological Cancer.* Pp. 99–103. Cardiff: Cardiff University Press.
DOI: https://doi.org/10.18573/book2.q. License: CC-BY-NC-ND 4.0

Hi Jac, it was called squamous carcinoma of the vulva. Other letters say micro invasive vulval carcinoma.

Squamous means to do with the skin, and carcinoma is the term for malignant tumour, so in lay terms this means that Becky was diagnosed with a tumour, or lesion, in the skin of her vulva. 'Micro invasive' means that a tumour measures less than two centimetres across and invades the skin to a depth of up to one millimetre. Quite small then, but hardly insignificant nonetheless and, because of the nature of the disease, these measurements can never be absolutely precise. In Becky's case the lesion was found to be invasive to a depth of approximately one and a half millimetres. Where vulval cancer and, indeed, cancers in general are 'staged' according to the severity and extent of the tumour, or lesion, Becky's cancer was not extensive. It would have been considered a Stage 1.

Although I have been doing a lot of research into the subject throughout the *Drawing Women's Cancer* project, it has to be noted that, clearly, I am not a medical doctor, nor have I any training in surgical procedure and so, although I may have misgivings about the extent of the surgery that Becky underwent given the size of her tumour, and although these misgivings continue to gnaw away at me with a hunger that reason cannot sate, they are founded only on speculation and concern, rather than on fact. I hasten to point out that medical decisions as to how to approach individual cases are based on more factors than simply the nature and stage of the disease, and I will leave my concerns there, still, albeit unquiet.

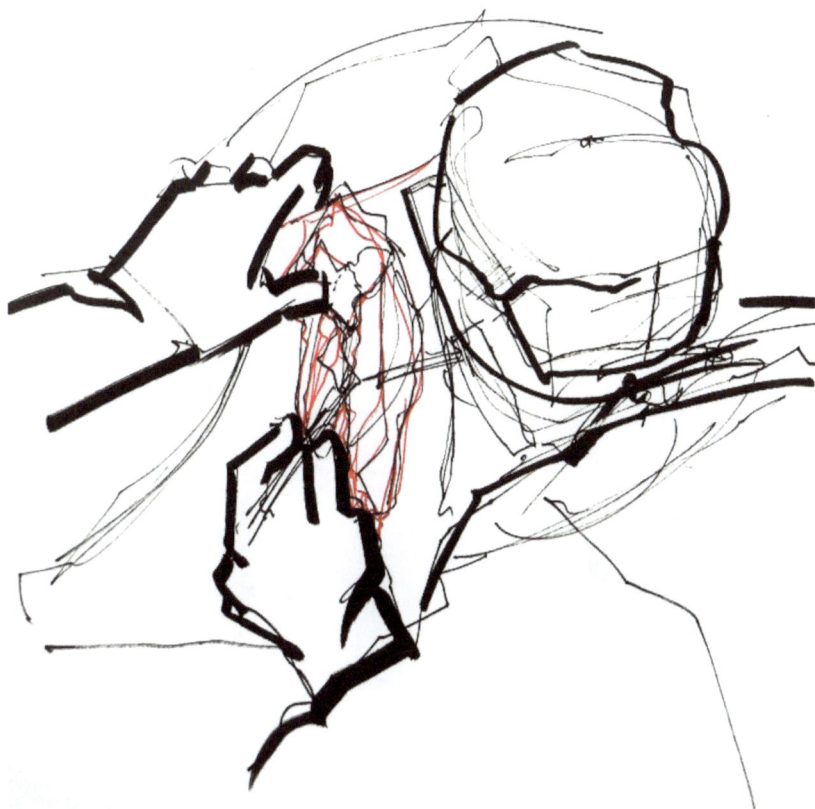

VULVAL SURGERY 1: *Ink on paper*

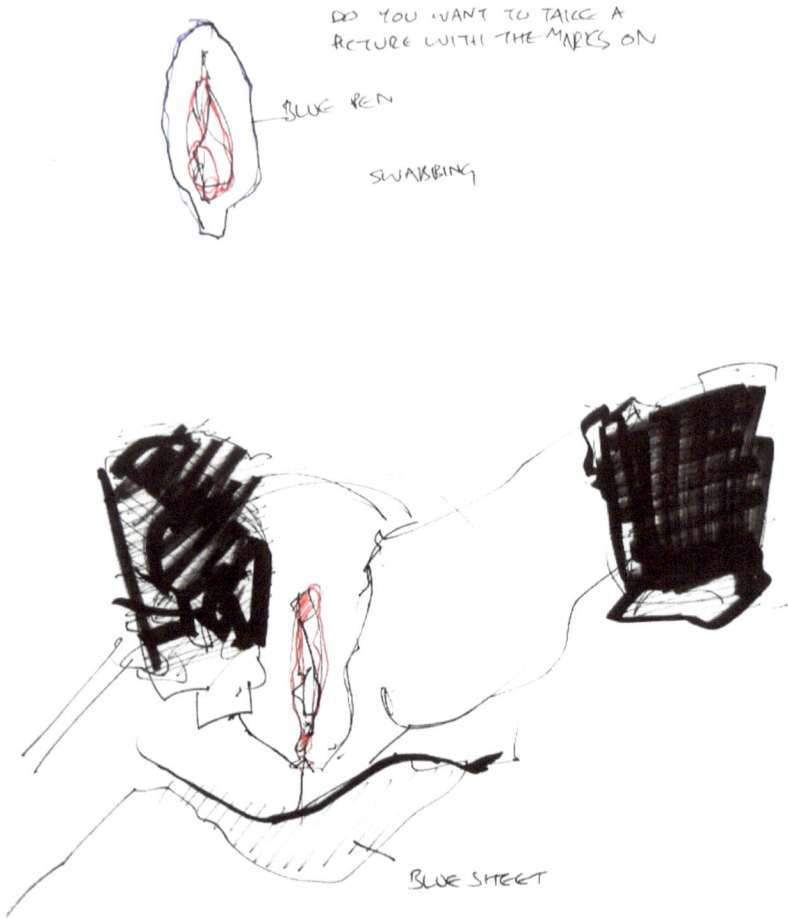

DO YOU WANT TO TAKE A
PICTURE WITH THE MARKS ON

BLUE PEN

SWABBING

BLUE SHEET

VULVAL SURGERY 6: *Ink on paper*

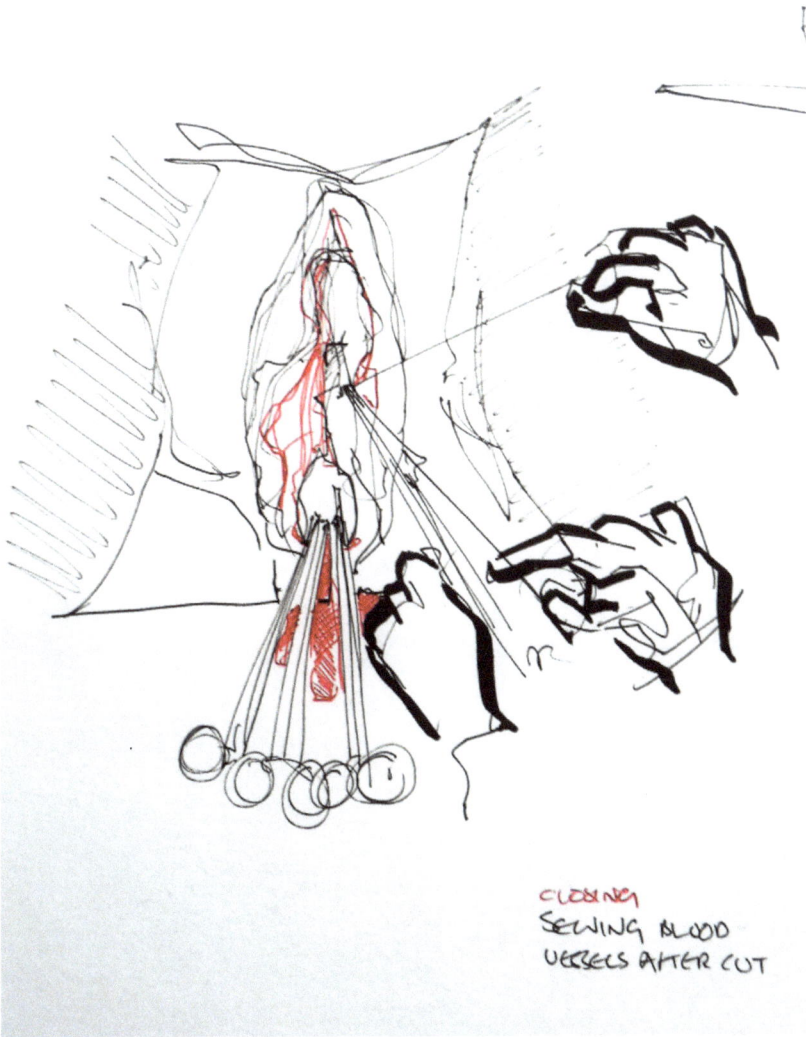

CLOSING
SEWING BLOOD
VESSELS AFTER CUT

VULVAL SURGERY 10: *Ink on paper*

I attended several operations during the *Drawing Women's Cancer* project and these three drawings are part of a series made rapidly in my sketchbook as I watched surgeons carry out vulval surgery.

If you love until it hurts, there can be no more hurt, only more love.

Mother Teresa

Becky. Return Visit: Part 6

The ten days I spent in hospital were hard. The day I came home after the operation Matthew gave me a beautiful Pandora bracelet. It made me feel special. Matthew and my parents looked lost and my brother didn't know what to say. I wanted things to be normal even though they were not. I wanted everyone to be normal around me. It was so good to be home, but I wasn't very mobile, I had to have a lot of help doing things like dressing and washing. Basically I couldn't do anything for myself and that was really tough for me to accept. Me and Matthew had to prepare ourselves; our life was going to change.

A few days after I got home my stoma nurse came to see me to check on my colostomy. The only question I had was, 'How long will the swelling take to go down?' She told me that it wouldn't go down at all because they had cut through the main muscle of my stomach and when I heard that I was gutted. I know it shouldn't have bothered me but it did. I couldn't get out much but when I did I had to go in a wheelchair and after two weeks I had to go back to see Dr T to get the results of the operation. I knew I had to get myself better as soon as I could because of the wedding. We were definitely not going to cancel. I had all sorts going through my head but some days I just sat and cried. I didn't know how I was feeling; it's so hard to describe it. Some days I felt as if I couldn't breathe.

My appointment with Dr T went really well. She told me that the operation was a success so I didn't have to have any chemotherapy and it was a relief. Now I could concentrate on getting better. I was missing work and the girls and I asked about my hen do. Dr T said it would it be ok to go as long as I was careful. Day by day I was getting used to my colostomy bag and getting to grips with fitting it properly. I would always have at least one a day that would leak though, and in the beginning that would really upset me.

How to cite this book chapter:
Saorsa, J. with Phillips, R. 2019. *Like Any Other Woman: The Lived Experience of Gynaecological Cancer.* Pp. 105–107. Cardiff: Cardiff University Press.
DOI: https://doi.org/10.18573/book2.r. License: CC-BY-NC-ND 4.0

The wedding was coming up fast and I decided I wanted to irrigate for two weeks before the wedding so I didn't have to worry about my colostomy bag filling up too quickly, especially with my wedding dress on. My stoma nurse came to the house to show me how to do it, but she only showed us once, we had to remember it all. I was a little paranoid about messing it up but Matthew was with me every step of the way and I remember the nurse saying that not many men would be so supportive.

Irrigation is a way of gaining some control over bowel function where the patient has a colostomy. It requires a plethora of equipment including a container for water, some tubing, a flow control/regulation clamp, a plastic cone, an irrigation sleeve and pegs, a disposal bag and some dry wipes. Matthew was indeed supportive over Becky's wish to carry out this procedure herself and, although she could most probably have managed it alone, Matthew was never prepared to let that happen. Even though helping his young bride-to-be with her colostomy irrigation can never have been a part of his agenda for the run-up to his marriage, he did so without complaint, and indeed with love. To demonstrate this, and before continuing with Becky's own words, I think it is fair to note in detail here the daily procedure that Matthew so willingly carried out for her.

With Becky sitting as comfortably as she could on the toilet, Matthew's first task was to connect all the irrigation equipment together – the container, the tubing, the cone, the sleeve and the regulator – and fill the container with lukewarm water. The amount of water to use always varies according to the individual and so it can be a bit 'trial and error' at first. The next step in the process was to remove the stoma pouch and make sure Becky's stoma itself was clean before he had to hold the water container above her shoulder while slowly opening the flow control clamp. Water had to initially flow into the tubing to remove any air that might have been trapped inside it. After this, and once he had closed the flow control clamp again, Matthew had to attach the irrigation sleeve to Becky's stoma, making sure the end of the sleeve was in the toilet. Then the cone, connected to the tubing, could now be gently inserted into the stoma through the opening at the top of the sleeve. While Becky held the cone in place, Matthew gradually opened the flow control clamp so the water could flow gently into the stoma, and, once the necessary amount of water had entered, he could remove the cone, roll up the sleeve over Becky's stoma and secure it with pegs. After about 30 minutes, when the sleeve was full, it could be rolled out and the end left in the toilet to empty. It could then be removed, put into the disposal bag and thrown away.

Every single morning at 8am for two weeks Matthew helped me irrigate. He almost drowned me a few times but we did it and best of all, on my wedding day I managed to walk down the aisle. I walked very slowly but

I did it. I could feel everyone's eyes on me but I focused on Matthew and when I got to him I could tell how much he liked my dress. He told me how beautiful I looked and that he wasn't expecting me to go for that kind of dress. He looked so smart and we were so proud.

Our honeymoon was already booked. We were going on a cruise around the Far East. I had another appointment with my oncologist in between the wedding and when we were supposed to be off and because she was happy with my progress, I was healing well after the operation, she said it would be OK for me to go, although I had to take my wheelchair because I still couldn't walk tidy. Meanwhile, Matthews back seemed to be improving. It was not perfect but we thought it was the best it was going to get. He was definitely looking better. Our honeymoon was fantastic, the break really done us good.

Sometimes, do you ever wish time stood still? A few months after the wedding I started to feel quite low. I didn't really know what was happening to me. My stoma nurse said that I might be depressed and she gave me a number for a place called Rowan Cancer Care where they have people you can talk to. So I phoned them and made an appointment with one of their counsellors.

Regaining my confidence was a nightmare, I just didn't know how to get it back, how to feel right again, but Matthew always tried to make me feel better. He was always telling me how beautiful I was. In the meantime Dr T was happy with the way everything was healing but my bum area was taking a bit longer than they thought so I had to wait to have my colostomy bag reversed. It wasn't so bad. It was part of me now and I was dealing with it OK. My belly still bothered me though because I felt like it was sticking out all the time. I had to have a few more operations to have more skin taken away to be tested. All the results but came back OK which was good of course but it was hard to go through one operation after another.

I finally had the colostomy reversal operation in May 2012. The weather outside was glorious. I was allowed home the following day and I was really sore. I couldn't do much again. It was so hard trying to walk around. I couldn't sleep tidy so I stayed on the couch for two weeks because it was hard even to get into bed.

Becky was not to know it at the time but this was the beginning of long-term suffering caused by chronic and unremitting pain.

The person who takes medicine must recover twice.
Once from the disease and once from the medicine.

William Osler

SUTURE 6: Kate. Endometrial Cancer

Diagnosed in May with endometrial cancer, Kate was referred from her local hospital for treatment in Cardiff, where now, on a sunny August morning in 2014, she is sitting up in bed on the Delyth Ward at the Cardiff Women's Clinic, calmly waiting to be taken down to theatre. It has been a worrying transition from spring to summer this year as Kate has travelled across the border between the two Kingdoms, of the Well and of the Sick. Now the operation to remove her womb is due to begin at noon, she is second on today's list, and I have come to be with her and bear witness. She has been expecting me and smiles as I enter the room. As she does so I notice that her greyish-blue eyes are bright and flecked with silver. They seem to dance in the harsh light of the ward as the smile lifts and lightens her face. Waif-like, her slender form makes only the smallest contour under the thin sheets, and as we shake hands I try to conceal my surprise at how small hers feels in mine.

Kate has come to Cardiff from Abergavenny, the hometown that she loves. She tells me that the referral to Cardiff concerned her initially, making her think that there must be something 'really wrong', and I try to reassure her that this is a worry I have heard a lot from patients who bypass their local hospitals and come to Cardiff for treatment. The reality is that their extra journey is not necessarily to do with the severity of their condition; it is rather that Cardiff, as the regional centre, is far better equipped and staffed to deal with complex oncological surgery than most local hospitals. Nevertheless, Kate's concerns only highlight an obvious need to give patients more information about their referrals, if only to avoid adding even more worries to the fear and confusion that many of them already feel.

As an enthusiastic participant in *Drawing Women's Cancer*, Kate tells me that she's seen the project website and that she has been reading the blog. She says that she thinks the work is 'really important'. I am very happy to hear this, of course, and I tell her so. The consent form that I am bound by protocol to offer

How to cite this book chapter:
Saorsa, J. with Phillips, R. 2019. *Like Any Other Woman: The Lived Experience of Gynaecological Cancer.* Pp. 109–123. Cardiff: Cardiff University Press.
DOI: https://doi.org/10.18573/book2.s. License: CC-BY-NC-ND 4.0

is on her bedside table and, seeing me notice it, Kate leans over to pick it up and hands it to me, saying, 'You see, I've signed it already for you.' I feel oddly embarrassed as I mutter a thank you before stuffing the form into a folder that I have in my bag. Such paperwork always seems to be an unhelpful interruption in situations like these, but I need to collect a signed form from every person I talk to in the hospital and, at the end of the day, I must deposit them in a drawer in the medical office, where they are kept secure. Ethical standards are important. I know. I must be seen to respect and adhere to them, not least because the future of the project depends on my doing so, even though the statutory and sometimes officious nature of such procedures usually, at least from my perspective, seem alien against the easy-going and trusting nature of genuine human relations.

Kate herself clearly suffers none of my misgivings about what, in the end, is a very small matter in the grand scheme of things, and her easy manner and generous smile invite me to relax. I smile back and move towards the large wingback chair that is next to her bed. Actually sitting down, however, proves to be quite a complex manoeuvre due to the distinct lack of space around the bed, and the chair itself being almost covered by the curtains pulled around the neighbouring cubicle where two nurses are attending to another patient. They are helping her, it seems, into a wheelchair, and the curtains, hanging loosely between the cubicles, do restrict our view but are themselves creating no physical barrier to an invasion, albeit unintentional, into Kate's already small area. And, just to add to the already somewhat bizarre situation, the patient being helped must be either deaf, or elderly, or both, as the nurses have to raise their voices almost to a shriek. It crosses my mind that, as Kate is very softly spoken, my recording of this meeting is going to make for an interesting transcription. Kate starts to giggle at my predicament and, shuffling over in the bed, she insists that I sit on the side of it. I do feel a little awkward but there's not much alternative, so I 'perch' on the end, just beyond the small triangular form under the sheet where her feet must be. I turn on the recorder and we begin.

She is still giggling as she obediently says her name into the recorder, but her smile wavers a little as she begins to talk and to recall the anxieties and the frustrations of recent months. She tells me about the numerous medical appointments that were scheduled at two-week intervals during what felt to her at the time like a painstakingly drawn out process towards her final diagnosis. But in the end, as Kate is keen to point out, the diagnosis itself came as less of a shock than it might have done, perhaps because of the protracted run-up to it. Of course, I am listening carefully to what Kate is saying, but I have a sense that there is more to this, and as she continues I soon discover why. She tells me in confidential tones about her pervasive feeling of strangeness about all that has happened since May because, she admits, she has feared having cancer for as long as she can remember. In confidential tones she says, 'Now that I actually have a diagnosis, weirdly, I feel better.' I say nothing. I feel she needs a little space so I simply nod to let her know I am listening carefully, while, for her, the paradoxical nature of her experience seems to come more into focus as her gaze slips momentarily beyond me and out into somewhere beyond the ward. I simply wait, in silence, as with this quiet shift of emotion she seems to escape from the current reality of the 'here and now', wherein her long-held fears have taken painful form, and go to somewhere else, a place perhaps where irrational feelings tend not to hurt so much. I wonder where that somewhere is, maybe where home is? The woodlands around Abergavenny? Wherever it is, it is certainly a long way from here, from me, from this small cubicle with the nurses behind the curtain still trying to manoeuvre the wheelchair and its confused occupant.

But she's not away for long; there's just enough time for a cloud to scurry across the sun and then she is back, shifting her own fear and confusion aside by telling me about how, since she has been ill, she has realised to her innocent surprise how many people around her either have or have had some type of cancer. 'You would never know!' Her sense of astonishment is grounded in almost palpable emotion, and indeed there is nothing disingenuous about her whole manner. She is smiling again, and I smile with her. As we talk, sometimes our smiles turn into laughter, and sometimes they give over to pain, but all the while I feel deeply moved by her generosity in allowing me to witness her confusion, her sense of disempowerment in the face of a situation she has always feared and now has to endure.

Kate wants to emphasise that she deliberately hasn't looked at any Internet sites for information about her condition because, as she says, 'I don't want to know'. Her apparent strength of conviction and purpose is mitigated however by her lowered eyes. It feels almost as if she is confessing some kind of misdeed, but when she looks up again there is no shame in her expression, only resilience and a calmness that seems to come from an implicit trust that everything will go well. But even if Kate herself doesn't surf the Internet she lets me know that her husband certainly does. She giggles again as she tells me how he logs on to relevant websites on a regular basis, and how ironic she feels it is that he has even signed up to a chat forum about endometrial cancer! Her love for her man is very clear as, with a wistful sigh, she tells me how he insists on giving her snippets of what the forum members are saying, and she is obviously thinking about him with fondness as we talk about the 'man thing', the way that husbands and partners in this situation often want to do something to 'fix' the problem. But we both understand, as indeed I have no doubt her husband understands, that the 'fixing' is not necessarily the real issue here; it's just that in the face of such emotional trials and crises we all have to do something, in our own way, to work through feelings and hurt.

Kate's way right now is to begin to talk to me about how she feels about her own body. It is obviously difficult for her and, as she does so, her voice becomes even quieter than before and I have to lean in a little in order to hear. It is as if the words themselves are causing her pain, and she leaves long silences between the phrases as she speaks. The nurses have now left the adjacent cubicle, pushing their elderly charge in her wheelchair, and there are no other patients on the ward. We are alone, and the silences weigh heavy on us both. Once again, an air of detachment comes over Kate, but this time the cloud over the sun is darker, heavier with tears. She is speaking slowly, softly, and, when she says 'I'm leaving all that to them', I make the assumption that 'them' signifies the medical team who are caring for her. As I listen, and she continues to talk about her feelings, Kate's detachment from the physical reality of her condition starts to make sense because she acknowledges that she is 'More concerned with what is going on emotionally, in my head'. She is obviously struggling to make sense herself of her feelings, to not let them take over, and indeed it does seem that she has succeeded, up to now at least, to defend herself from her own emotions, albeit at some cost.

But time has moved on, a fact emphasised here in the ward by the loud ticking of the clock on the wall, and Kate begins to talk about the impending operation. She says that she is most worried about how she will actually recover and is almost apologetic as she admits that 'It is hard. It actually *hurts* to know that, although I'm feeling fine right now, no symptoms as such, I fully expect to go home feeling much worse than when I came in here.' I can only nod to show that I understand because, however much I want to reassure her, deny her fears, tell her she will be fine, I cannot. We both know that she is right. We both know that next few months are going to be very difficult, because while recovering from major surgery she will also be undergoing the chemotherapy that she has been told by the medical team is a necessary follow-up treatment. But she has a goal! She suddenly looks directly at me and her smile, now returned to light up her face, is even broader. She says, 'I walked up Pen y Fan the other day in the glorious sunshine. I'm going to do it again, before Christmas.'

Empathy here is too academic a word, a concept, for what I am feeling. I want so much for her to walk up that damn hill, and I want to tell her that she will, but I cannot because I know that nothing can be so certain. I would never lie or even fudge the truth just to placate someone, just to make them (or would it be even to make myself?) feel better, especially someone so honest and so genuine as Kate. It comforts me to imagine that neither would she ever really expect me to, so we talk instead about the project, about the need for more communication about gynaecological cancer and about how women need themselves to talk about their experiences, just as she is doing now. We talk for what seems like a long time, but as the idea of the operation becomes increasingly real Kate becomes visibly upset. She tells me about her family – 'I have three sons' – and as she does so she places both hands very gently on her stomach. 'It's where they were created.' Then there are tears. I reach for her hand and we smile for each other. I say, 'Some things don't need to be said.' She nods.

We do not talk so much about the details of the procedure she is about to undergo, except to acknowledge her relief that, because the operation will be a laparoscopy, at least she will not have to undergo open surgery. Neither do I mention my mixed feelings in anticipation of my first time witnessing this 'keyhole' method. I am actually surprised at the excitement and expectation I feel, but at the same time I am concerned as to whether this reaction is somehow inappropriate and, inwardly chiding myself because my 'dilemma' really is far less important than how Kate herself is feeling, I direct my thoughts towards how to take my leave without feeling as if I am abandoning her. The clock on the wall ticks on, mercilessly, and Kate becomes thoughtful. 'You need to go. Prepare for theatre.' She smiles as I hesitate. She says, 'I'll be fine.' I smile back, not sure who she is reassuring the most: herself or me.

The operation

The treatment for endometrial cancer is a full hysterectomy, that is, the complete removal of the womb. Often this involves making a large incision in the patient's abdomen, either vertically from navel to pubic bone or laterally across the bikini line. Either way this is a huge operation that inevitably leaves a long scar. Fortunately, in Kate's case her tumour is well defined, which means that she can therefore have a far less invasive procedure, a laparoscopy, commonly known as 'keyhole surgery'. A laparoscopy is performed by the surgeon 'remotely', using handheld, long-shafted instruments that are inserted into the patient's abdomen through very small incisions that leave minimal scarring. The two main advantages of this kind of surgery over the more invasive operation are that the smaller incisions reduce the risk involved in potential blood loss during the operation, and they lessen the time it takes for the patient to heal and recover.

The primary instrument used in a conventional, or 'cold-stick', laparoscopy is the laparoscope itself. This is a telescopic rod lens system that is connected to a tiny video camera and a fibre-optic 'cold' light source, either halogen or xenon, which relays images of the inside of the abdomen or pelvis to a television monitor above the operating table. The surgeon works alongside an assistant, who is responsible for positioning the laparoscope correctly so that the surgeon can see images on the screen of the inside of the patient's body, and those images will guide the way that she works. Further instruments are inserted through three or four separate small incisions in order to perform the operation. This form of laparoscopy is indirect in the sense that, while she is working from images on the screen, the surgeon is not actually looking at the real patient lying on the table, nor does she the see the real, physical part of the patient's body that she is operating on because the incisions are only made large enough to accommodate the slender instruments she is using. There is therefore a level of disconnect between surgeon and patient but not so much as in the case of robotic surgery, where the operation can be performed by a surgeon who is not necessarily even in the same room.

Two surgeons, Dr M and Dr J, will perform the operation, and I take advantage of the chance to chat with them before it begins. It is music to my ears when Dr J, while eating his salad lunch from a plastic Tupperware carton, tells me that his choice to specialise in obstetrics and gynaecology was in major part based on his belief in the benefits of real communication with his patients. He says that in his experience of other areas of surgery there is not so much emphasis on a supportive role, on talking with patients about their diagnoses and about their treatment, but in 'obs and gynae' he has found more opportunity to offer what he calls the 'personal touch'. So here is a surgeon who wants to talk to his patients, and as he talks to me it is clear how much he has internalised and understands the import of a subjective perspective, even in situations where he has to, necessarily, maintain objectivity. Indeed, doesn't the sheer physicality of what a surgeon must do demand emotional subservience, a level of professional detachment, intellect over sentiment? Who after all would want a surgeon who is operating on them to be anything less than totally focused on the job at hand, objectively? But subservience need not be synonymous with inertia; on the contrary, it seems to me that emotion, compassion and human understanding can only serve, when under sufficient control, to strengthen the will, hone the intellect and steady the hand.

Just on noon I gently knock and enter the 'green room', the operating theatre where Kate's procedure is due to take place. Four surgeons are bent over a patient who is comatose on the operating table, her belly open and bloody. Everybody acknowledges my presence with a smile; even the surgeons look up from their work, and I feel welcome. I am a familiar figure now in theatre, quietly moving around in the background with sketchbook in hand, making sure to avoid getting in anyone's way. The patient on the table is a large woman. From the glimpse I get of her face, partially covered as it is by the oxygen mask she is wearing, I can see that she is much older than Kate. She must be the patient scheduled before Kate, the first patient on today's list. The theatre nurse sees my confusion and comes over to let me know that the operation has become far more complex than was first anticipated and is taking much longer to complete. Kate's procedure will be delayed. I am tempted to stay now I am here, but I know I cannot. This patient has not consented to being part of the project, and so I take my leave, respectfully, and as I am in scrubs and cannot go back to the ward I go the office instead, to wait. I feel a pang of sympathy for Kate as I imagine her still waiting in her cubicle, and I hope that someone has let her know why she has not yet been brought down to theatre.

Two hours later, Kate's inert body is finally wheeled into theatre. She looks so small and slight on the bed, even smaller than when she was under the covers on the ward, and so very vulnerable. I feel strangely at odds with myself because I cannot quite identify how I feel on seeing her here, unconscious and oblivious to all the activity around her. Maybe it comes from what she said earlier about leaving her body up to the doctors. Maybe I feel protective. I have to continually sidestep, backwards and forwards, to make sure I stay out of the way of the nurses and technicians who are hurriedly setting up equipment for the operation. Their preparations are so confidently and artfully carried out, with everybody seeming to know exactly what they need to do, to my untrained eye it looks as if the whole thing is choreographed. It is a complex 'dance', a form of well-ordered chaos, and unlike anything that I have seen before. The efficiency is impressive and I feel, very keenly, the shortcomings in this environment of my qualitative roots, transplanted as they are here into a quantitative soil. My own subjectivity and that of Kate, lying peacefully now on the table and covered with green sterile cloths, seems almost irrelevant now because here, in this room, in this theatre full of science and instruments, objectivity steps up to the front of stage, to take its accolade, and I can 'feel' the fame of it. I *want* to understand everything, but I *know* I never can so I try to focus on the things that will stick in my mind. I make some sketches but mainly just watch in awe.

As well as the permanent video screen in the corner of the room, two more screens are being positioned around the operating table, along with their accompanying gadgetry. Powerful lights are set into place and sterile instruments are counted out, noted on the whiteboard and laid in order on the table that is positioned directly beside where the surgeons will be working. As the technicians move everything into place and set up the scene, the surgeons, the principal actors, are in the small room at the back of the theatre, preparing to play their parts. I can hear them laughing and chatting about things that are way beyond the small, separate world that this room has become as they scrub their hands, don gloves and masks, and pull cotton caps over their hair. The anaesthetist keeps his vigil at the head of the bed, checking his data as Kate breathes softly beside him, her greyish-blue eyes now softly closed and the lids held down with tape. Finally everything is ready.

Dr J draws up a low stool and seats himself at the end of the table, between Kate's legs, which are now raised in stirrups and spread apart. He needs to position a plastic 'device' into her vagina, before carefully suturing it onto her cervix at the neck of her womb. He tells me that the device will provide a hard surface to cut onto when the operation is under way. The device is a bright green colour; later it will become startlingly luminous on the screen. Both surgeons are now standing either side of Kate, and a junior doctor takes Dr J's position between her legs. The green cloths are folded back to expose her abdomen, which is anointed with iodine. It is then filled, 'insufflated', with carbon dioxide gas to such an extent that her belly swells to become grossly disproportionate to her slight frame and, poignantly, resembles a pregnancy. Dr J tells me that the expansion elevates Kate's abdominal wall to create a space above her internal organs. This allows him to see, very clearly via the laparoscopic camera, the area that he needs to work within. Carbon dioxide gas is used because it is common to the human body. It can be absorbed by tissue and removed through Kate's exhalation as her breathing is controlled and monitored. Importantly, and reassuringly, carbon dioxide is also non-flammable, an obvious asset where electrosurgical devices are being used.

Working together, and with immense concentration, Dr J and Dr M insert four separate instruments into Kate's abdomen, into the space expanded by the gas. The incisions through which the laparoscopic camera, the two 'grippers' and a diatherm are introduced are tiny. The diatherm is the same instrument – albeit on a smaller scale – as the one I watched being used throughout Tracey's hysterectomy. Dr J reaches up to make minor adjustments to the position of the video screens and the two surgeons begin to work. Physically detached from what they are actually doing inside Kate's body, their hands do control the instruments, but at an arm's length, and the reality, the actual mechanics of all the searching and the cutting, is only visible on the screens above. It is as if they are playing a video game, watching images that continuously change and move with a concentration that is extraordinary to witness. This is hand–eye co-ordination tested to its limit.

My pen hangs idly in my fingers. My sketchbook remains closed. I cannot draw. I am transfixed by the screens. Cut, cut, seal, cut. A multitude of images flitting in cinematic abandon whenever Dr M or Dr J moves the slender rod that holds the camera inside Kate's body. They need to 'delimit the anatomical target area'. The colours of the separate organs are translucent, like the oil glazes that I use when I am painting. They move seamlessly over each other as the steel instruments begin to invade, just as the glaze moves over the scumble at the stroke of a brush over canvas. As I watch the diatherm ruthlessly dissecting the boundaries between tissue and hue, the imagery on the screen becomes almost hypnotic as art and science coincide and colours coalesce into a kaleidoscope of tonal value that favours every nuance, and none.

Despite myself, I cannot help thinking about colour, and my concentration wavers. In terms of the art–science relation, which is indeed a fundamental driving force in the *Drawing Women's Cancer* project as a whole, colour itself can be understood as a fundamental linkage between the two. The power that colour has in bringing art and science together, a power that is almost tangible here in the operating theatre, comes perhaps in part from what Johannes Itten calls its 'beauty and immanent presence'. The indication of religious fervour in Itten's protestations about his subject lacks subtlety, and it is made even plainer as he goes on to assure us that you have to love colour before it will unveil its 'deeper mysteries', but, as a leading figure of the Bauhaus, Itten himself strad- dled the boundary between subjectivity and objectivity, demonstrating that artists are certainly not the only ones to be moved by the guile of both nature's hues and their synthetic counterparts. Itten aside, as an artist, the 'mystery' of colour resides for me not so much in the practical use I put it to, and cer- tainly not in any scientific or even religious understanding of it. For me, colour demands a philosophical perspective. According to John Gage in *Colour and Meaning: Art, Science and Symbolism* (2000), author Stephen Melville may well have felt the same as he at least posed the philosophical problem of colour even though he neglected to actually address it. But *how* to address without encoun- tering grey areas? Derek Jarman wrote about grey as the 'sad world into which colours fall', Kandinsky's grey is 'void of resonance', combinations of colours when mixed without care on the palette will move towards grey, so Melville's colour, for colour's sake, must remain:

> Bottomlessly resistant to nomination, attaching itself absolutely to its own specificity ... even as it appears subject to endless alteration arising through its juxtaposition with other colours. Subjective and objective, physically fixed and culturally constructed, absolutely proper and end-lessly displaced, colour can appear as an unthinkable scandal.

Kate's eyes are grey. Greyish blue.

I fight my way back from my musings and, watching the continuing invasion of Kate's internal organs as they flicker across the screen, I begin to feel disorien-tated within the 'unthinkable scandal'. The transition from living form to two-dimensional video screen is confusing. My understanding of what I am seeing becomes lost in the communicative space between and I struggle to recognise even which way round I am actually seeing the organs that are being highlighted, silhouetted in transparent colour, in flat form. But, suddenly, all becomes clear in the 'champagne layer', the soft veil of bubbles, caused by the gas, that float, sparkle and gently explode into tiny fingers of light inside the artificially inflated cavity that is Kate's abdomen. The surgeons smile at my involuntary gasp as I watch Kate's fallopian ligaments finally take comprehensible form, just before they are separated and mercilessly severed. Now her uterus, the womb that car-ried and nurtured her two sons, hangs forlornly between the ovaries, its broad ligament like the outstretched wings of a weak and dying bird, trapped, exposed and inevitably vulnerable to predation. So much detail, so many metaphors, so much association and yet so many disassociations.

In Kate's abdominal cavity her blood begins to pool in smaller hollows and fissures between organs. On the screen it pulses with the deepest and richest of red hues, opaquely defying the colourful translucency of the surrounding tis-sues. But the blood is 'excess'; it obscures the surgeon's view and is a hindrance to the work. A rich life source has now become merely an inconvenience for the meticulous procedure being carried out and so it must be sucked out through a flexible tube, wasted, spent. In the clarity it leaves behind, the surgeons can locate the ligaments that secure the uterus to the body, and they neatly sever them. Kate's womb, along with the cancer that invaded it, finally succumbs to being cut out by its very root.

Chemotherapy

After her operation Kate had to undergo a course of radiotherapy followed by eight cycles of chemotherapy at Velindre Hospital in Cardiff. Just as she was happy to talk to me and be part of the *Drawing Women's Cancer* project from the beginning, she readily agreed to meet up with me again to talk about her experiences. All of the arrangements were made via email.

16 Sep 2014 17:36

Hello Jac

I've just returned from Velindre and my radiotherapy is due to start next week – Monday to Friday at 11.30. How are you placed? Wednesday would be a good day for me as I have some time before I have to be in Brecon for 2.30.

Then I'll be back at Velindre on 30th for the chemo planning day which I gather involves a lot of hanging around with periodic blood tests, so that could be another possibility, though it may be difficult for me to get into the centre of Cardiff between blood tests (and I see what you mean about the 'busyness' of Velindre – though there's always the car!)

17 Sep 2014 10:39

Hi Kate

Very glad to hear from you and also that you have finally got the dates sorted out for your therapy. Wednesday works for me… you are most welcome to come to The Broadway of course but I am happy to meet you at Velindre if it is easier/preferable for you. It is busy yes, but then I need not record our conversation – simply make notes afterwards.

I am free also on the 30th… just in case you have to be there alone and might want some company to 'hang around' with!

Let me know what you think

Jac

18 Sep 2014 10.08

Hi Jac

Shall we say this Wednesday? I'll get back to you after I've been tomorrow when I should have a clearer idea of when Wednesday's session is likely to finish. Would it be OK for you to come to Velindre?

22 Sep 2014 21:30

Hi Jac

I should be finished by 12.00 on Wednesday. I don't know how busy it gets at that time, but P and I went to a very quiet cafe before my appointment this morning and were the only people there – the Roundabout cafe (on the roundabout!) next to, and attached to, the Methodist church. I just wondered whether that might be a suitable place to meet up?

As I walk to the Roundabout Café near Velindre Hospital in Cardiff I feel the last remnant of warmth from an elderly summer sun on my shoulders. The tree-lined street is bright but the leaves shine gold and bronze in the cool light. The year is in decline. Kate and her husband are already at the café, sitting quietly in the corner drinking coffee. She smiles and rises, carefully, from her seat as she sees me come in. As I approach she leans towards her husband and something passes between them that I don't hear, then, after a brief introduction and a warm handshake, he politely takes his leave. He does not go far, just to the other side of the café. He finds a seat and pulls a newspaper from his bag.

I buy myself a coffee at the counter. Kate is still going on with hers, and she and I settle down to chat. There was no recording equipment this time, just us, chatting. She looks a little tired but otherwise remarkably well. Something is different, though, and then I notice that her hair is shorter than before. 'It looks good,' I say, and Kate smiles ruefully. 'I'm preparing for the chemo. I know it's going to fall out so I thought I might as well make sure there'll be less to clear up!'

The conversation gets to a deeper level very quickly. Kate doesn't want to talk about the radiotherapy itself; for her it is more about the certain knowledge that both it and the chemotherapy that is to follow will make her feel a lot worse before it makes her feel better. It is a similar feeling as she had expressed in the hospital, when we met for the first time, and I feel as inadequate now as I had done then in trying to find an answer that would make even the slightest difference. But Kate doesn't seem to notice. She asks about the operation, keen to know how it was for me to witness it. So I tell her about how the colours and the images were almost overwhelming. I tell her that the whole experience was for me profoundly emotional both in my concern for her as the patient but also, and I had to admit it, in relation to my sense of self as an artist, confronted by the majesty of the human body in all its colour and beauty and light. I tell her that I stood in awe of the professionalism of the surgeons, of the skill, the efficiency and, yes, the care that they showed in the way that they opened her to minimal view yet were able to carry out what needed to be done. I tell her too about an exhibition of artwork that I will be putting up in November, and she says she would like to come. I tell her about the narrative I am writing about her operation (this narrative), and she says she would like to read it. She listens patiently to everything I say. She smiles and seems to enjoy, to share my enthusiasm. She says she wishes that she could have seen the images on the screen as I did, even though it feels odd to her that we are actually talking about her own body. She says she is glad that the project is happening and that she can be part of it.

After an hour or so Kate's husband folds up his newspaper and returns to the table. Kate and I are laughing about something silly. Since the first rush of words we have been talking about anything, everything, except cancer. It was good to talk, she says, good to take her mind away from the treatment and its consequences, at least for a while. Her husband looks concerned as he takes her hand. We part, promising each other to, of course, stay in touch.

7 Oct 2014 15:34

Hi Kate

I hope that things are going as OK as they can be… the chemo has begun?

I am working on the text and will send it on as soon as I have the draft complete.

My thoughts are with you

Jac

15 Oct 2014 09:44

Hi Jac

Thank you for your message, and apologies for not getting back to you sooner, but we've been without Internet for the past week (rather blissful in its own way!), and I'm only now able to catch up.

The chemo went well with just the expected tiredness, apart from a rather angry rash that appeared the day after the treatment and a temperature, the combination of which put me in our local hospital overnight. They treated it as shingles though I don't think they knew for sure. That aside I feel remarkably well, so fingers crossed the next and subsequent sessions go OK.

It was good to see you again, and I shall look forward to seeing the piece you have written about my op in due course. How are preparations for the exhibition coming on?

All best wishes

Kate

16 Oct 2014 11:38

Hi Kate

Thanks for your email. Its good to hear that you are managing the chemo well, although the rash thing sounds nasty. Hopefully it will be a one off and things will be smoother next time.

The show is coming together… I am trying not to panic too much about it! I understand of course that you cannot make the opening but hopefully you might feel well enough to come see it during the week – with you husband too of course.

As promised I am attaching the piece I am writing re your op. It is a rough draft and naturally I would appreciate any comments you may have and of course any changes you would want before putting up on site. For instance, I have used your real name in the piece but of course

I can make it anonymous… just, whenever you are ready, let me know what you think.

All best then and take care

Jac

19 Oct 2014 18:53

Hi Jac

Thanks for sending the piece about my operation. It is fascinating to read what went on – I'm sorry to have missed it! I'm happy with what you say, and for you to use my actual name. Where is it intended to be published? You probably did tell me, but I've forgotten? (Pen y Fan with F, by the way).

Yes, P and I are hoping to get down to the exhibition – we'll have to play it by ear as to when's the best time.

Good luck with it

All the best, Kate

21 Oct 2014 09:38

Hi Kate

So very glad you are happy with the piece (and thanks for the spell check!) I want to put it up initially on the *Drawing Women's Cancer* site (drawingcancer.wordpress.com) but I will use it eventually however as part of the book I am working on re the project as a whole.

It would be really good to see you both at the show – it goes on till Sunday 2nd so just let me know whenever you will be able to come and I will be sure to be there.

See you soon then…and take good care

Jac

26 Oct 2014 17:50

Hi Jac

Hope the private view went well and we're sorry not to have been able to make it – I had a seven-hour chemo session on Friday, so didn't feel much like trekking down to Cardiff. However P and I would like to come next weekend and I'm wondering what the gallery's opening hours are??

Looking forward to seeing the exhibition…

Best, Kate

26 Oct 2014 19.03

Hi Kate

Seven hours! That's a lot to take… I hope the side effects this time are not as harsh as before.

Friday night went very well thanks. Unfortunately I will be teaching on Saturday and on Sunday afternoon so the time to come would be Sunday morning or, even better would be during this week if that were possible for you. I really hope you can make it.

Best wishes

Jac

Kate's husband came to the gallery in Cardiff later that week. Kate felt too ill to make it. The exhibition was entitled *Illness begins with 'I'* and he seemed fascinated, as I accompanied him around the show, by the images that spoke mostly of illness and the more painful aspects of the human condition. He bought a small, framed drawing. An elderly lady, suffering. I wrapped it very carefully.

6 Feb 2015 16:22

Hi Kate

I hope you are doing OK and getting over the Chemo.

As I will soon be off to Glasgow University for three months of writing up the *Drawing Women's Cancer* project you and all the women I have worked with are very much in my thoughts. I want to say then thanks very much again for your patience and generosity in being a part of the project.

I will be posting on the blog again throughout my time up there so you may be interested in seeing how it goes.

All best wishes

Jac

8 Feb 2015 12:52

Hi Jac

It's now two weeks since my final chemo (fingers crossed). I've been fine through it all, but successive treatments have knocked me back, so I'm pleased to have finished.

It's all been a bit hectic, as I've been trying to organise our kitchen refurbishment at the same time – not a good idea with a 'chemo brain', as I've found it really difficult to make decisions and then stick to them!!

I do wish you all the very best as you continue with the project in Glasgow. I really hope that your project will help raise awareness of women's cancers – I've found it extremely useful just to be able to talk to you about it. So thank you.

I shall look forward to following your progress on the blog.

With all best wishes

Kate

9 Jul 2015 22:15

Hi Jac

I'm feeling well, and have resumed 'normal' life – whatever that is! And my hair has come back curly!

I shall look forward to following your activities on your blog.

With all best wishes

Kate

10 Jul 2015 08.41

Hi Kate

Curly hair eh! I am sure that it suits you very well!

All the very best to you both

Jac

A drawing is not necessarily academic because it is thorough, but only because it is dead. Neither is a drawing necessarily academic because it is done in what is called a conventional style, any more than it is good because it is done in an unconventional style. The test is whether it has life and conveys genuine feeling.

Harold Speed

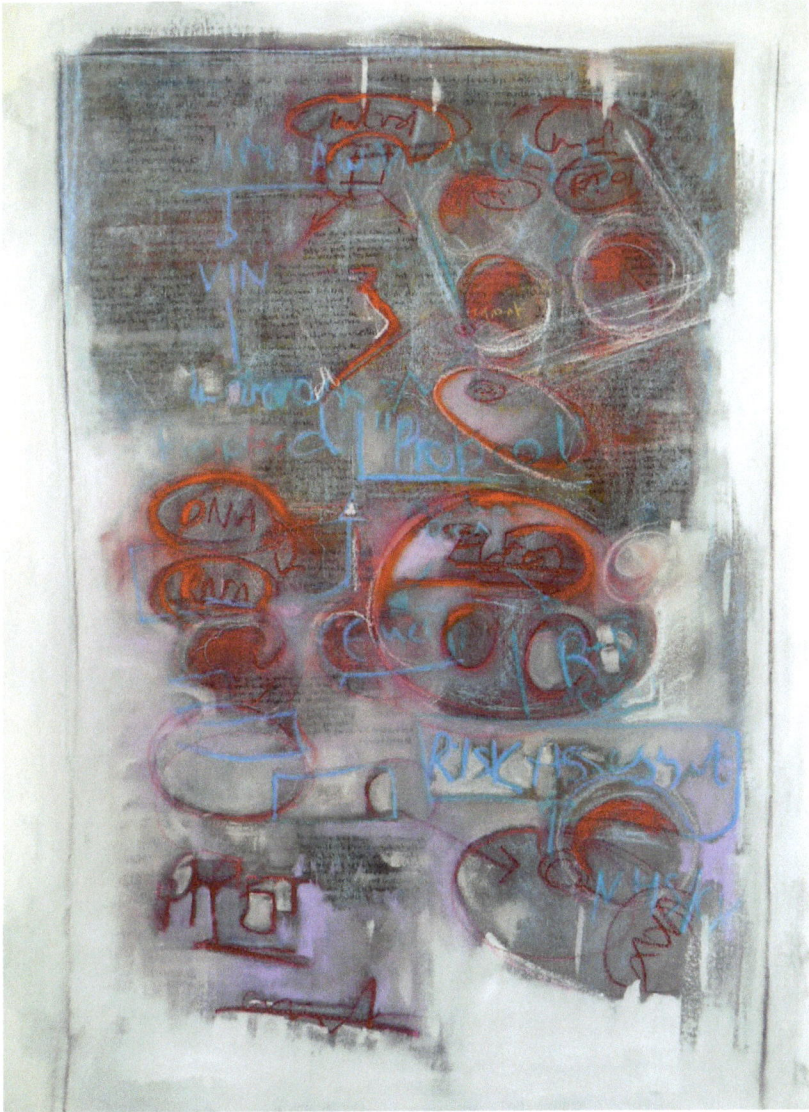

NOTES: *oil paint, chalk, pastel and ink on canvas with oil ground*

This piece represents the importance of language both conventional and visual. Elements of the transcripts from my conversations with women patients and with medical staff are here overlaid with drawings that are copies of the diagrams drawn for me by the surgeon as she explained operation procedures.

Becky. Return Visit: Part 7

To be honest I felt worse after this operation [the colostomy reversal] than after any of them and after a few weeks I began to feel this horrible pain in my belly. I didn't know what it was and as time went by the pain was got worse it was frightening me.

Fear of the unknown and its accompanying terror of the possibilities is always mentally and physically debilitating, and in Becky's case it is only compounded by the suffering she's already been through in the aftermath of several operations besides the original major surgery. Sitting now before me, she looks small and vulnerable, bolstered by cushions on her comfortable sofa in her warm home while the rain starts to come down again in earnest so that its pattering on the window creates a tearful soundtrack. In that embarrassingly verbal fumble that often ensues from an awkward silence we both begin to speak at the same time. 'Please,' I say. 'After you.' But her pretty face begins to crumple with emotion as she describes the extraordinary and chronic pain that she has been suffering over the past months, the cause of which none of the medical team seem able to identify.

I've been three times in hospital... I thought I was dying, that's how bad the pain is... it frightens me. I've had scans and everything... the pain is coming from where my colostomy scar is and sometimes it's so bad I don't know what to do with myself. It even makes me vomit. The last time I was taken into hospital the doctors referred me to the chronic pain doctors. I've got pregabalin tablets and I have steroid injections every three months but nothing is working. I've had this pain constantly now. I went back to see my counsellor because my mood keeps getting real low again.

How to cite this book chapter:
Saorsa, J. with Phillips, R. 2019. *Like Any Other Woman: The Lived Experience of Gynaecological Cancer.* Pp. 127–130. Cardiff: Cardiff University Press.
DOI: https://doi.org/10.18573/book2.t. License: CC-BY-NC-ND 4.0

Becky pauses, as if the all the explaining has been too much for her. I can see that things are not right and all the optimism that she must have had once the original surgery was completed has since seemed to fade away. Again, I begin to say something but Becky starts before me. The timeframe has shifted back now as she is describing an operation she had in the time between our first meeting and now.

> I'm still back and forth seeing the gynaecologist and every six months I see my plastic surgeon as well. I noticed where they'd removed the skin from my bum area it had dropped. It was like… well, it was on the top of my legs so Dr D wanted to redo it. I wanted it done too. It was like having a bum lift! So he put me on his waiting list he told me I would only wait about three months.

I realise that this must be the operation that she had come to discuss with Dr D on the day that she and I met at the women's clinic, well over a year ago now. That was the day that he was unable to see her and she was happy to talk with me so that at least her long journey to the hospital had not been a waste. Naturally she wrote about the operation in her notebooks:

> *When it was time for the operation the plastic surgeon drew on my bum to show me what he was going to do. It looked good to me. He told me I would be in hospital just for the one night. Everything went well and when I came round I had drainages in the tops of my legs and my bum was really sore. Matthew and my mam were waiting for me on the ward as usual. In the morning Dr D came to see me and to have a look at the cuts. He was happy with everything so the drainages could come out, fresh bandages put on and then I could go home. I had to travel for an hour in the car and that was unbearable, like I was being injected, or cut with knives.*

Besides the pain she is clearly suffering, the foremost issue on Becky's mind is still about getting pregnant and becoming a mother. As much as she wants it, Becky is conflicted, worried, and only naturally so in the circumstances, about her abilities to be a 'proper mam' at all. 'When I have a baby I want to be able to enjoy it; I don't want to be in pain all the time.' Her ambivalence is founded on genuine concerns, and as she talks about it I begin to berate myself for betraying the unaffected authenticity of what she is saying by feeling sympathy for her rather than an equally genuine empathy. I wonder why, or perhaps what, I am holding back, and I hope that it is simply my own 'stuff' and that it doesn't show, that Becky cannot sense anything wrong.

The doctors have told Becky that the physical changes to her body during pregnancy *may* abate the pain, at least for the nine months, and the possibility of this, however remote, seems to be an idea that she is hanging on to, one that is at least comforting, if not reassuring. Freedom from pain and the chance to become a mother are all she really wants and her expression softens even at the thought of them. But there is of course no certainty. None to say that pregnancy actually would alleviate the pain, and none to say that she could even become pregnant in the first place. Moreover, even if she were to conceive and carry the child to full term, she knows too that because of the scar tissue she would have to undergo yet more surgery because of having to have a caesarean section, which of course would leave her with 'another scar I've got to deal with'.

Becky asks me if I have children myself. I feel strangely self-conscious and even vaguely guilty as I confirm that I do, but as she looks me directly in the eye I can also feel the dogged determination that has clearly been a part of her ability to deal with all that has happened to her. Now she says, simply, 'I do want to have a baby,' and I just nod as a tacit agreement is forged between us.

There is another short silence but this time it doesn't feel so awkward. It feels rather as if both of us have descended into a labyrinth of thoughts and emotions around the idea of motherhood in general. For myself, my sense of family suddenly becomes very real, almost tangible. My own two children, now grown into beautiful and inspiring adults, suddenly seem very close even though both are living their individual lives at a distance. My mind begins to drift as I think of my daughter, who favours the sun and lives, sporadically, in warmer climes across the globe, where she dives in crystal-clear waters trying to find something she has long been looking for. Her brother, my son, is still here in the rain. A fine musician and songwriter, he peers deep into the soul, without flinching, and expresses what he sees there through evocative sound. I am thinking about how much being a mother means to me, about how much Becky deserves the chance to also be a mother, and about how she would undoubtedly be a good one. Such a simple need, a natural wish, but how much and how effectively it is complicated by the repercussions of all she has gone through. Oddly, perhaps, I am also wondering about whether she would ever consider adoption, either in the worst scenario of her not being able to conceive or as an alternative to undergoing yet more surgery on her already scarred and, let's be honest, somewhat mutilated body. But I chide myself for such thoughts, try to push them aside and inwardly tell myself that this is about Becky and her perspective on her own situation, nothing to do with my own opinions or any detached rationale. And so, despite any misgivings I may have, or worries for Becky's health were she to get pregnant, I can totally understand, in my head and in my heart and without her having to say any more, how much becoming a mother would mean to her and, most importantly, how much she would willingly go through in order to achieve it.

Just as I am struggling with my own muddled ideas, and perhaps feeling the weight of the past few moments, Becky delves into my thoughts and lifts them, along with the conversation, up and out of the past and into possibility. There is a wistfulness in her tone and in her expression that resonates with a lighter future where more than simply the wish for a child is at stake. She smiles as she says, 'It would be nice to go back to a bit of normality.'

Normality. The day-to-day mundanity that for her is perhaps the most profound loss of all and, even as she thinks on this and despite her attempt to lighten the mood, the very word, normality, seems to become a weight that once again bears down on her. She is speaking more slowly this time, vulnerable and unsure of herself. 'Every day that I'm in pain… I know it's a bit extreme but some days it gets so bad I could literally just get into the car and drive into a wall… and I'd think… it doesn't get any easier. I don't feel sorry for myself… I dunno… it's just difficult.'

I am trying hard not to 'jump in' here, not to offer what could only become empty platitudes, inappropriate and ineffective, destined to be tossed about on the surface of the ebb and flow of her thoughts. Empathy is what she needs. An attempt to understand what is underneath and behind the words that she uses to describe a pain that we both know can never be fully contained, in either a physical or an emotional context. She begins to tell me about a photograph she has. It is on her dressing table in her bedroom and she looks at it every day. The photograph is of herself with her girlfriends, all dressed up for a night out, and it was taken just three months before her original diagnosis. As I listen, conjuring up pictures of my own of the carefree group, Becky's voice wanes and her gaze seems to turn in on itself, as if she is visiting, no, not just visiting, *reliving* the past. Just for a fleeting moment she is obviously unaware of my presence as a multitude of emotions cross her face. I see, in quick and random succession, vulnerability, fear, regret and a frown that admits of the acute sense of unfairness that she must strive, every day, to control.

Then she is back in the room, with me. She smiles. A brave face. 'God!' she says. 'What would I do to go back. On a night out. Just to get dressed up and… I felt good about myself then. Just to go back… to have just that one day of feeling normal like being able to bend when I want to. I didn't think twice about bending.' Again, I say nothing. What is there to say? I just nod and hope that she understands how much I care. She seems to. I tell myself that the trust she has in me is clear in the way that she is being so open in telling me how she feels. Recently, she says, she has had an appointment with the genetics department. She has been suffering tenderness in her breast. There is a strong incidence of breast cancer in the immediate family and she is to start mammograms, even at her young age.

As a family we spoke about getting genetic testing done but we only spoke about it at first. A few weeks later I had a pain in my breast. I knew there wasn't anything serious wrong but with the family history my mother wanted me to go to the doctor to get it checked out. The doctor asked me about any family history of breast cancer and when I told him how much there was he suggested that we go through genetic testing, he kind of set us thinking again. When we told my Nan what we were going to do I don't know if she felt happy about it she didn't say much and every time we brought it up in conversation she always changed the subject. She was afraid.

It is not despair,
for despair is only for those who see the end beyond all doubt.
We do not.

J.R.R. Tolkien

The Miscarriage

In the years since our meeting at her house in late 2013, Becky has been through many trials, most due to the ongoing chronic pain that she continues to experience. Just a few months after that meeting, however, something happened that was to affect her fundamentally and test both her resolve and her fiercely held sense of optimism to the limit. For the next part of this narrative, the focus will be primarily on her story, as written in her own words. At the time of writing it is summer 2018, but to step forward we must at the same time step back.

It was the summer of 2014 and in August we had some very exciting news. I found out that I was pregnant! I can't even tell you how we were feeling it was amazing. The only thing I was concerned about was how I was going to be with my pain but it didn't matter because I would go through fire and water to have a baby so even if it meant I had to stay in bed for nine months I would do it. This felt like our reward for everything that has happened to us, and it was nice to have some good news for a change.

I know a lot of people wait until their twelve-week scan before they tell anyone but we couldn't keep it to ourselves. My mam was at home with us to and when I shouted it out she began crying. I couldn't believe it myself until I went to the doctors and it was all confirmed. Sometimes I would pinch myself to make sure it wasn't a dream. I had an appointment with Dr W. They wanted to keep a close eye on me because of the vulval cancer and I already knew that I wouldn't be able to have a natural birth because of the reconstruction. My skin just wouldn't stretch that far. I was feeling a bit rotten, sick and tired all the time, but I wasn't moaning.

On the day of my appointment, in the waiting area there were pregnant women everywhere. I was around nine weeks pregnant. The nurse called me in and Matthew and my mother came with me to listen while Dr W went through a few things, and then he wanted me to have a scan so he could have a look. We were so excited. I got up on the couch and Dr W put jelly

How to cite this book chapter:
Saorsa, J. with Phillips, R. 2019. *Like Any Other Woman: The Lived Experience of Gynaecological Cancer.* Pp. 133–135. Cardiff: Cardiff University Press.
DOI: https://doi.org/10.18573/book2.u. License: CC-BY-NC-ND 4.0

on my belly and he was being really gentle because of my pain. He couldn't see that clear so he said he would need to give me an internal examination so that he could see better. He said to Matthew 'hold her hand', and then he told me that it was twins... but there were no heartbeats.

I couldn't talk. I felt like someone had ripped my own heart out I couldn't catch my breath. I had to get out of there. I couldn't understand why. I hadn't had any bleeding but my babies were dead and all I wanted to do was curl up into a ball. Something that we had wanted so bad had been taken from me. Why?

When we got home I got straight into the bath and I lay there looking at my belly hoping and praying that the doctor may be wrong. I knew deep down he wasn't but I had to hold on to that little bit of hope. That night I lay on the couch with Matthew and cried like I couldn't stop. Matthew was trying so hard to be strong for me but it felt like there was one horrible thing after another and there was nothing I could do about it. We were looking for answers but there weren't any, it was just one of those things that happens, but I still began to think, was there something that maybe I did wrong? I was on what felt like a slippery slope down and I didn't know how I would come back from this. I didn't sleep a wink that night. I just lay awake thinking about what could have gone wrong.

The following morning the hospital rang to say I had to have another scan done and because it had to be at the antenatal I really didn't want to go. But I had to go and this time the scan was much clearer. I could see them inside me and it was heart wrenching. Matthew and my mother, the both of them were crying and it was horrible. After the scan I had to go up to ward five to see what the next step was going to be. The nurses were really nice, but I really didn't want to be there, and they had to explain that I had to take a tablet and go back to hospital two days later. They told me I could start miscarrying in the house, and if I did they wanted me to try to recover what I lost so that they could see it. I felt so very bad and it felt wrong. The next two days were a blur I didn't speak a lot. We just couldn't get our heads around what was going on. Nothing happened in the house so I returned to the hospital where the next procedure would happen. I had to have another tablet, inserted this time, and wait. The nurses were already aware of my chronic pain so I had plenty of pain relief as well as gas and air.

It had been almost two hours and nothing was happening so I had to take another tablet. Then the pain came on real strong and nothing would ease it. The gas and air helped a little but I was so sad. I can't remember the things I said but I can remember Matthew and my Mam crying, especially Matthew, he found it very difficult seeing me like that. Then an hour or so after the second tablet things started happening and, Oh, it was horrific! No woman should have to go through that. The nurses had a look at what

I had passed and they were happy for me to go home. They wanted me back though in fourteen days so that they could check my hormone levels.

We got home round eight in the evening and that night, and for many weeks after, I cried myself to sleep. Matthew would wake up, and hearing me cry, he would give me the biggest cwtch ever. He always did whatever he could to make me feel better. It was another tough time and even though I was so glad I had Matthew and my parents, I got really low. I didn't want to go out and I knew in myself that it was time to go back to see my counsellor, just to try and get myself back on track. I booked an appointment with Hayley a week after I lost the babies and when I got to see her she knew something awful had happened. It helped to talk to her about everything. This was the first time Hayley had seen me cry.

She suggested something that could help me to accept what had happened. A memory box. I thought that is a good idea. Over the next few days I started to gather things that made me and Matthew happy, like photos, special birthday presents, just little things that made us smile, and I wrote a letter to my babies. I knew they were in safe hands because my two nans were looking after them. During the next few weeks when both my brother's girlfriend and my brother-in-law's wife found out they were pregnant I was so happy for them but, I'm not going to lie, it did hurt too.

I went for my next appointment to check my hormone levels and I had to have a blood test exactly two weeks after that. When I rang the hospital to find out what the results were, unfortunately they showed that my hormone levels hadn't come down so I had to go back again a week later. I think my hormone levels were still high because I hadn't actually lost everything, so I had to have another ultra sound scan. This was so hard for me and it went on for weeks. I had to keep going back to the hospital and each time it got harder. I couldn't even try to move on because I was constantly reminded of what happened. Every so often I would sit on my bed and get our memory box out just to have a look. This helped me.

The greatest hazard of all, losing one's self, can occur very quietly in the world, as if it were nothing at all.

Søren Kierkegaard

SUTURE 7: Maria. Ovarian Cancer

Maria was diagnosed in 2006 with ovarian cancer and she underwent a hysterectomy. Now a biopsy has shown a recurrence where the cancer has metastised into her bowel, and there is also cancer in her left breast. She requires a 'left breast procedure', another name for a mastectomy, and a 'debulking' operation on the tumour in her bowel. At 48 years old, Maria is a full-time carer for her husband, who has heart disease. She therefore wants to get her own health issues 'over with quickly' so that she can continue to look after him. She has insisted then on having both procedures carried out in one operation so as to reduce the number of times she'll need to be in surgery.

Even from my layperson's perspective, Maria's decision to undergo two forms of major surgery in a single procedure seems drastic and, while talking with the surgeon, I wonder aloud how much advice she'd been offered. The surgeon herself expresses some concern but shrugs her shoulders as she confirms that Maria has insisted. The immensely complex operation is therefore set to go ahead this hot July afternoon. I decide to take a walk in the sunshine, just to collect my thoughts and try to separate them from my misgivings.

A little later I return to the ward to meet with Maria before she goes to theatre. She has agreed to take part in the *Drawing Women's Cancer* project and for me to be present during her operation, and I am anxious to at least say hello before I witness the huge ordeal she is about to undergo. But she is asleep. I do not want to disturb her. I quietly leave, only hoping that I will see her awake later on after everything has been a success.

Now dressed in blue scrubs and with sketchbook in hand, I perform my usual dance around the operating theatre, moving backwards and forwards and side-stepping to ensure I am not in the way of people and equipment as the scene is set for Maria's anaesthetised entrance. She is next door, counting down from 10 as she passes into induced unconsciousness. But there are delays. The usual

How to cite this book chapter:
Saorsa, J. with Phillips, R. 2019. *Like Any Other Woman: The Lived Experience of Gynaecological Cancer.* Pp. 137–141. Cardiff: Cardiff University Press.
DOI: https://doi.org/10.18573/book2.v. License: CC-BY-NC-ND 4.0

fluid efficiency I have come to expect in these rooms is today compromised by a systems failure. The anaesthetist's equipment isn't working properly and a lot of time passes as the technical problems are sorted out. I am wondering where and how Maria is during all this. Is she still waiting behind the swing doors? Still sleeping under the influence of something more than the exhaustion she has been feeling over the past months of illness? The surgeons complete the paperwork as technicians battle with the equipment. It is noted that Maria is allergic to penicillin.

Finally Maria is wheeled into theatre, her inert body lying peacefully supine on the trolley. Four people heave her onto the operating table and, as she lies for a moment illuminated in her vulnerability under the harsh light, it is as if her humanity, naked and raw, is powerless against a tide of objectivism. I sketch her image into my book, rapidly, hardly lifting the pen from the page. I have to be quick in order to capture something of her person as in a matter of moments theatre staff are covering her with green, sterile cloths, leaving only the parts of her body that are to be operated on exposed. They are chatting as they work and, when they are done, Maria has become an object to be opened, manipulated. The anaesthetist has more care, more sensitivity. As he takes his place at Maria's head, continuously checking his equipment, the look of concern and frustration that he wore earlier dissolves and softens into one of concentration and composure. He bears a huge responsibility for his charge and his compassion shows as, gently and thoughtfully, he puts out a hand to stroke a stray hair from Maria's forehead as she breathes softly and steadily into the mask that covers her face.

There are now 11 people in the room. Three teams of surgeons will be working on Maria, one for the mastectomy and two others for gynaecological and colorectal procedures. The breast surgeon will begin and already the theatre nurses are brushing Maria's exposed left breast with iodine until it is covered entirely and is the colour of molasses. The breast surgeon is brusque in manner, almost aggressive. I know a few of the surgeons now through my work in this hospital, but this man is not someone I've met before. He seems impatient, irritable, and only mutters his name during the ritual round of introductions. He barely acknowledges my presence in the room, and I have the sense that he does not approve of my being there, but once the operation begins he is clearly focused entirely on the work he is doing, despite anything else going on around him.

The surgery begins with the stripping away of the thick yellow fat that adheres to the taught skin encompassing the large, flaccid preponderance that is Maria's breast. The surgeon is working with two assistants, junior doctors who seem in awe of their mentor, and so three pairs of hands are carrying out this delicate work, cutting, stripping and holding back the breast itself from its own surface. The initial cut through the skin is triangular in shape. It is not something I have seen done before in the other mastectomies that I've witnessed. In those, the surgeon always made a straight cut, bisecting the nipple. Here however there are two diagonal cuts and the nipple remains intact at the apex. I am confused and I make a mental note to ask about the technique once that operation is over.

The mastectomy is completed cleanly and efficiently in a very short time and, seemingly, with no problems. Maria remains sleeping peacefully under the anaesthetist's watchful eye. Her chest, now quite lopsided, still rises and falls gently and easily. Meanwhile, the room, which had been reasonably quiet, now bursts into life as the nurses and auxiliary staff scurry about organising the equipment for the next part of the procedure. I need to be quick on my feet to stay out of everybody's way and I manage to make some hurried sketches of Maria on the table with a myriad of tubes and wires extending both from and to her.

Dr K, a surgeon I know well, now steps forward to begin the debulking operation. I interviewed him about his work very early on in the project and now, as I watch him make a long vertical cut that opens Maria's abdomen from the costal arch to the pubic bone, I remember him telling me that he had always known he would specialise in obstetrics and gynaecology, even as a first-year student in medical school. He is a softly spoken man who exudes patience and understanding. He obviously cares deeply and likes to talk with and get to know his patients as individual people, rather than them being just another on his list. I imagine that he inspires a lot of confidence in his patients, but the juxtaposition of this with seeing him now, performing such a dramatic and visually brutal invasion into Maria's unconscious body, makes me feel just a little bit disorientated. With the cut made, special clamps are set to hold open the wound while Dr K and another surgeon, now working calmly and efficiently, lift out and sift through Maria's intestines with their gloved hands. Watching from a couple of feet away it is difficult for me to distinguish the bloodied flesh from the bloodied gloves and the bloodied cotton swabs that they are using to mop up the excess bodily fluids. There seems to be red everywhere. It changes the green cloths brown and stains the cuffs of the surgeons' white cotton coats, increasingly so as the sifting through Maria's intestines continues. It seems to take a very long time, but eventually they locate the primary tumour, a hard, white mass in the red, and they take a specimen for analysis. After replacing her innards the surgeons now need to locate Maria's urethra. They find it quickly and use a sling to isolate it, make it safe from harm, ready for the next surgical team to begin cutting away more of the tumour. Then we wait. The next team is still working on another patient. Maria continues to breathe steadily and peacefully. Her belly, now wide open, is covered with only a thin layer of gauze, and as I wait I watch, transfixed, as her blood gradually diffuses across the gauze and it begins to stiffen and take on a deep ruby hue. Eventually the conscientious theatre nurse replaces it with a fresh piece, and the staining begins anew.

After around 30 minutes another surgeon enters the theatre. A colorectal specialist, he *is* the next 'team'. He comes in confidently, enthusiastically, greeting us all with a cheerful smile and offering profuse apologies for being 'so behind'. A tall slim man with a very educated English accent and turn of phrase, he seems oddly out of place, but he is clearly very good at what he does, judging by the level of respect he seems to command from the others and which is now present, almost tangible, in the room. It seems to hang in the air, rendering mute any discontent that may have been building up in his absence.

Without further overtures the newcomer begins to work on Maria's passive form with Dr K and the other surgeon assisting. It surprises me that the three of them are talking between themselves, as if the rest of us are not here, about social lives and other things totally unrelated to the job in hand while at the same time they are delving and probing into Maria's abdomen. They continue to pull aside her intestines in order to locate and cut out large parts of the malignant tumour that is lurking there in the depths, debulking it in order to ensure that the consequent chemotherapy and/or radiotherapy that she will need will be as effective as possible. Debulking is a specific procedure that is used only in malignancies where the tumour is too large to remove in its entirety without damaging surrounding structures. Sadly, this is the case for Maria. It is usually a long and complicated procedure and, as I watch, the effort begins to show on the faces of the surgeons. They cease to banter between themselves and a heavy silence descends on the whole room, interrupted only by the noise of the equipment and occasional demands from one or other of the surgeons for a scalpel, a probe or suchlike. The theatre nurse is efficient and attentive with a supply of sterilised tools constantly at the ready.

Witnessing this scene of controlled carnage before me I am reminded of something that Dr K said during my conversation with him about his work several months ago. The talk had turned to gardening, bizarrely, perhaps, but on the other hand he was explaining to me the ways in which he managed to relax, to 'come down' and free himself at least temporarily of the tensions and anxieties around patients and procedures that were a significant part of his chosen profession. Yet, even in an activity supposed to take him away from the stresses of his job, he finds something that relates. He says:

> The thing [about gardening] that relates very well to what I do is when I have to get a tree root out. It means that you have to go down digging, find the source and take it out slowly bit by bit. But it is only the persistent gynaecologists who go in and take things out because you have to spend a long time. You have to get the cancer out. You may be slowly moving in from the outside so as to extract everything. You need to work your way out slowly. You need to get every last tendril.

Eventually, once the surgeons have agreed that they have taken out as much of the tumour as they safely can, all three of them begin to push Maria's intestines, which had been lifted out during the operation and left lying in a tangled heap on her belly, back into her body through the gaping wound. Dr K says, under his breath and almost inaudibly, 'We need to get them back in the same kind of orientation,' and I cannot help but marvel over how these vital organs can be shoved around, seemingly so casually. Finally, the Englishman, having done his work, exits the room as confidently and as much without ceremony as he entered some two hours ago. Dr K and his colleague are left to stitch Maria's gaping abdomen back together.

Postscript

During the wait for the English surgeon I managed to talk with the breast surgeon about his technique. I find out that it is one he has designed himself with the possible future needs of his patients in mind. The triangular cut is intended to create a scar that forms a 'ridge' on the rib cage where the fold of the breast once was. The ridge would then provide either support for a prosthetic, or, if the patient requested a reconstruction, it would make that procedure easier to carry out. I was impressed with the sensitivity of this surgeon, who has clearly thought about the feelings and practicalities for his patient, even though his brusque, almost dismissive manner might belie such a thoughtful approach.

Post-postscript

Maria got through the operation, which was deemed successful in both parts. However, she suffered greatly in the aftermath, with many complications setting in.

*Suffering is a fierce, bestial thing, common-
place, uncalled for, natural as air.*

*It is intangible; no one can grasp it or fight
against it; it dwells in time.*

It is the same thing as time.

Cesare Pavese

Becky. Searching for the Cause of Pain

After the miscarriage Becky was left in an emotional vacuum, and the chronic pain she was suffering, which, as she told me, 'Goes through my stomach, into my side, down my left leg and into my back', was still as intense. After reaching several 'dead-ends' on the circuitous route through NHS treatment, she took it upon herself to take control of the situation and find someone who could really help her. The search took her out of the Welsh NHS jurisdiction and into England. A consultant in Bristol finally confirmed that her pain was caused by nerve damage resulting from the colostomy reversal operation and, for Becky, finding out that there is indeed a very real problem eased to some extent her mental suffering. She was at least able to retrieve some sense of control over her own body and her own sense of self belief, control that she felt she had lost somewhere along the line.

As the weeks went by I began to feel better. I was going to see Hayley every week and she said she could see an improvement in me. But my pain wasn't helping and I was feeling very low. Nothing the doctors were trying was working, not even tablets. I used a hot water bottle constantly but now my belly is so badly burnt because I didn't realise how hot the bottles were, only that the warmth helped the pain. I felt like I couldn't cope with all this any longer so I started searching for a doctor that could help me. I searched for about nine months in total before I came across someone, a consultant plastic surgeon specialising in cosmetic and nerve surgery. His name was Dr M. I read about him and what I found out made me think straight away that this doctor could help me. I got in touch with his secretary. Her name is Mary. She is a very nice lady she ended up going above and beyond for me and I was so grateful. In that first call I practically begged her to make an appointment for me to see Dr M and although she did explain that he may not be able to help, I just wanted to see what he thought. I had to try something. There was an appointment available

How to cite this book chapter:
Saorsa, J. with Phillips, R. 2019. *Like Any Other Woman: The Lived Experience of Gynaecological Cancer.* Pp. 143–145. Cardiff: Cardiff University Press.
DOI: https://doi.org/10.18573/book2.w. License: CC-BY-NC-ND 4.0

for the following week and because I had to go to the Bristol Spire hospital Matthew arranged a day of work so that he could take me.

I was feeling excited to see the doctor and I was hoping that he could shed some light on what was going on with my pain. People were asking me if we were going to try for another baby, but the fear of something terrible happening again frightened me so much and my head still wasn't in the right place to try again. I had to give myself a bit of time especially as one of the hardest things was that none of the doctors I had been seeing were really sure what would happen with my pain if I were to get pregnant again.

It took us about an hour to get there and I was trying not to get my hopes up to much just in case he couldn't help me, but when he called me from the waiting area and introduced himself I thought to myself straight away what a nice doctor, he was very down to earth. He explained that he may not be able to help but that he would certainly try and that was good enough for me. He examined the area and he told me straight away that he thought my pain was nerve damage from having the colostomy reversal because my pain was centred right in my scar area. He said there were a few things we could try and that an operation would be up to me, but with him being a private doctor these things don't come cheap. I had a few appointments with Dr M after that first one and he tried some things to make the pain better but none of them worked so in the end he wanted me to go back to see my GP and get a referral to see him on the NHS in Stanmore hospital. I took it that this would be quite easy to do and I was feeling a bit overwhelmed because it seemed like I was getting somewhere. I knew it was going to take some time but I had to try to be patient.

I made an appointment with my GP so that I could get the referral that Dr M asked for but my doctor explained to me it wasn't going to be easy and that it would take a few weeks at least even to get an answer. I was so disappointed. I don't really understand the NHS sometimes because I couldn't find a doctor in Wales that could help me but I found one in England and then Wales wouldn't refer me straight away because of the cost. I also had a funny feeling the health board was going to refuse me anyway. I heard nothing for weeks and the worry of it was getting to me. In the mean time I was still trying steroid injections to ease the pain but they still weren't working and I just didn't know what to do. Finally I had a phone call from my doctor to tell me the health board had refused to pay for me to have treatment in England and I was so gutted. I couldn't hold back the tears because everything was going wrong again and I really felt no one was listening to me.

A few days later I decided to ring the Health Board myself, but to be honest I didn't really get a lot of information from the person I spoke to, they weren't helpful at all. So I got in touch with Dr M's secretary, Mary, to explain everything to her about what's been going on. I don't think Mary really understood either, why the Health Board had refused me, and so she did everything in her power to try and help me. I think that she really felt for me. She made another appointment for me with Dr M to see what else I could do and he suggested another doctor, Dr B, who was based in Swansea. Dr M said he wasn't one hundred per cent sure that this doctor could help me, but it was worth a try.

When I got home I did some phoning around. I eventually I got Dr B's secretary's number but when I finally managed to get hold of her she explained to me his waiting time was eighteen months! I couldn't believe what I was hearing and I asked her briefly about private work. She told me that the doctor works in the Spire hospital in Cardiff. I got off the phone and rang Spire hospital straight away. I managed to get an appointment with him in two weeks. From eighteen months to two weeks, just because its private! But there was no way I could wait eighteen months to see him.

Becky. The BRCA Gene: Part 1

While all this was going on the women in the family all finally decided to go through with genetic testing to see if we were carrying the BRCA gene.

BRCA1 and BRCA2 are two examples of genes that raise your cancer risk if they become altered. Having a variant BRCA gene greatly increases a woman's chance of developing cancer in the breast and in the ovaries.

We had to be taken through the process first to make sure everyone was making the right decision. My Aunt, Mam's sister did the test first because she had already had breast cancer. She was diagnosed thirteen years ago with stage three cancer, but she got through it after intensive chemotherapy and radiotherapy. She lost all her hair but she came out of it OK in the end. She had test done almost straight away at the GP surgery but the genetics doctor warned her that it would take a few months for the results to come back. In the end they took so long that she had to phone the surgery to make sure she hadn't been forgotten, and even then it still took some more time, but eventually her results came back. They said that she did carry the BRCA2 gene, even though she had got through the cancer, and this meant that my mother should definitely get tested. The doctor said Mam's results would only take about two weeks to come back, 'because they already knew what they were looking for.'

I could see that Mam was nervous about the results but she tried not to show it. I think that she already knew she carried the gene but while we waited for her results I was hoping and praying she didn't. I even kind of convinced myself she didn't but after two weeks we were back at the hospital and I went in the room with her whilst my aunt and uncle, Mam's brother, sat waiting outside. Dr R told my mother straight away. He said 'I'm awfully sorry but you do carry the gene', and I burst into tears because

How to cite this book chapter:
Saorsa, J. with Phillips, R. 2019. *Like Any Other Woman: The Lived Experience of Gynaecological Cancer.* Pp. 147–149. Cardiff: Cardiff University Press. DOI: https://doi.org/10.18573/book2.x. License: CC-BY-NC-ND 4.0

I had really made myself believe that she wouldn't have it. Dr R explained all the options about reducing her risks of cancer. First there was a hysterectomy, and then if she chose it, a full mastectomy. My mother had some very big decisions to make.

Even before we came out of the room I had decided to get tested as well. My Mother had already said she didn't want me to but I needed to know either way. Dr R made me an appointment for a month's time.

I was still trying to get something done for my pain but I wasn't getting anywhere fast. Sometimes I felt no one was listening. I had this appointment with Dr B but I really didn't want to get my hopes up at all because I really didn't know what to expect. When the day of my appointment finally arrived I didn't know how I felt to be honest. I told him everything, right from the beginning, and then, after he examined me he told me that although the operation would be possible it wouldn't be straight forward as it was more complicated than he thought. He said that he could give me only a fifty per cent chance of the operation working and that was disappointing of course but I was determined to go ahead. He said the operation could be done on the NHS, so that at least was good news, but he told me also to be a little patient because he had to get a team of doctors together to discuss what they are going to do. I left the hospital feeling happy and even excited.

Between going backwards and forwards to hospitals about my pain it was time for my genetics blood test to be done. My GP had a few problems getting the blood, I seem to never want to part with it, but he told me I would have to wait about four weeks for the results. It was fine with me, just another waiting game. Besides I didn't really think about it too much as, although I know it sounds stupid now, at that time the BRCA gene was the least of my worries. My mother was worried though. She didn't say much but I can read her like a book and I know when something is bothering her. I knew that if I found out I carried the gene I would somehow deal with it then, no point in worrying about what I didn't know, but still I couldn't get my mothers results out of my head. I suppose I was worried over her like she was over me.

I didn't wait long to have an appointment with Dr B. It was only a few weeks before I had a letter to go and meet the team of doctors who were going to operate. I was really hopeful. Just maybe this would be when things would start to look up for us. In the meantime though the results of my genetic text came in. They were positive. I do carry the gene.

I was there on time for my appointment at Swansea Hospital but I had to wait because the group of doctors I was meant to see were running a little late. It was only about twenty minutes but it seemed like longer as I was a bit nervous. I didn't know what they were going to say. Eventually I was called in and there were six doctors in the room. They all examined me and they all had their different inputs into what they were going to do in the operation. They wanted to try something there and then. They gave me an injection into the corner of my colostomy reversal scar, with a bit of local anaesthetic, just to see if that helped any with my pain, but it didn't touch me, it didn't do anything. Then they wanted to put an injection into my leg and that worked a little but my leg suddenly felt really weird. It was numb for a few hours after, but it soon wore off. The doctors told me I would be waiting about three months for the operation, which I thought wasn't too bad. I was on a high. I was feeling so much better just thinking that I was finally getting somewhere.

After that appointment I kept ringing the hospital, almost every day, to see if they had a date for my operation, but they kept on telling me the dates haven't come out yet so there was no chance of me having the operation before Christmas. It was disappointing but I tried not to let it get me down. Then, a few weeks before Christmas I began feeling unwell, more unwell than usual. My pain was still there of course but this was something different. For a long time, after all the operations, I suffer now with indigestion and heartburn really badly. I would get it in waves and it would last for some weeks and then settle, but this time it wasn't settling down. I was going backwards and forwards to the doctors to see why it was so bad and I had more blood tests and more tablets to take but this time my doctor referred me to have a camera put down my throat to have a look at what's going on. My GP told me I was a complicated patient, nothing was ever straight forward, but we had a giggle about it and he always says that he can't help the way I was formed in my mother's womb. He's a good doctor though. He put me down as urgent for the camera appointment but in the meantime he asked me for a stool sample. I took it down the following day and began another wait for results. They came back just a week before Christmas and they showed that I had H Pylori, a bacterial infection in my stomach. No wonder I was feeling so rotten.

Helicobacter pylori (*H. pylori*) is a type of bacterium that infects the stomach, usually during childhood. It is a common cause of peptic ulcers and, although it may be present in more than half of the entire world population, the majority of people don't realise they are infected because they never experience adverse symptoms. Where symptoms do occur, such as an ache or burning pain in the abdomen that is often worse when the stomach is empty, nausea, loss of appetite, bloating and/or unintentional weight loss, the infection can be treated with antibiotics.

The doctor gave me very strong antibiotics to take, which was really bad news because I knew from having them before that they made me feel sick and left a disgusting taste in my mouth. Even so I had to have them, and all over Christmas too! That was fun. As they started to kick in I began to feel better but my appetite had disappeared. The weight just dropped off me and I lost around three and a half stone.

The world breaks every one and afterward many are strong at the broken places.

Ernest Hemingway

Becky. The Nerve

Christmas came and went and 2016 came around. I know it sounds odd to be so excited about having an operation but I couldn't wait for it to happen, as I am sure that anybody, if they were in so much pain as I was, would do anything to try to make it better. I was impatient but I waited until the middle of January before I rang the hospital again. They still couldn't give me a date and I was really disappointed, but they told me to keep on ringing. Finally I rang Dr B's secretary to try to find out what was going on and she told me I wasn't even on Dr B's waiting list! She said that I was on another doctor's list, but nobody had contacted me to tell me that so by this point I didn't really know what was going on at all. She explained to me that if I wanted Dr B to do my operation I would have to wait around two years, and she also told me that my operation was now down as a normal routine procedure so it was unlikely that I would have an appointment any time soon. I was really angry because the doctors themselves had told me that the operation would be very complicated to do, so there didn't seem to be anything routine about it. I was starting to lose faith in the NHS. I felt like my problems were being ignored and I was getting brushed onto any doctor. I rang around and got the number for the secretary of the doctor whose list I was now supposed to be on, only for her to tell me that he was off work sick, and that he had been since the previous November. She also said that she didn't know when he was going to be back in work and she thought that it could be weeks or even months.

It felt like my heart was broken. I was so upset. I rang Matthew to tell him but I could hardly speak. It was happening again, I was taken two steps forward and five back, I was on a high and then straight away I was back down on a low. I couldn't take this anymore so I rang Mary, Dr M's secretary, and explained to her what was going on she could tell how low I was and I said I'd rung her for a bit of advice because I didn't know what

How to cite this book chapter:
Saorsa, J. with Phillips, R. 2019. *Like Any Other Woman: The Lived Experience of Gynaecological Cancer.* Pp. 151–154. Cardiff: Cardiff University Press. DOI: https://doi.org/10.18573/book2.y. License: CC-BY-NC-ND 4.0

else to do. The only thing I could think of was to pay for the operation, I wasn't sure how, but it seemed like it was the only option I had left, but there was another problem. Margaret told me that Dr M was not very keen to do the operation privately because he knew there was only a fifty per cent chance of it being a success and he didn't want me paying out lots of money if it wasn't going to work. I could understand that but I felt so desperate and Mary could tell that. She told me to leave it with her because she was meeting Dr M for lunch. I think she was going to have a chat with him about my situation. Very soon after Mary rang me back to tell me Dr M had agreed to do the operation and he wanted to see me to discuss the situation. I knew that I would have to pay for him to do it privately, and that was a worry, but I was over the moon. I had a smile from ear to ear and I was so grateful to Mary for doing what she did for me because she helped me as much as she possibly could. There are not a lot of people out there like that.

I did make a few complaints to the NHS because I felt that the way that they had treated me wasn't good enough, and I was hurt over the fact I had been put onto another doctor's waiting list without even being told. I received letters of apology but they didn't really help at all. In the end I was glad that I'd found Dr M and I think that what ever you want in life, if you don't go out and get it yourself nobody is going to do it for you. And, it's a good job we don't know what's round the corner, because if we did nobody would ever leave their houses.

I had the operation in February 2016. I went into hospital early in the morning on the day even though I was booked to go to the theatre at 2:15 in the afternoon. Different nurses and doctors kept coming backwards and forwards all morning while I waited in my room, they had to do all their checks. When it was time to go to theatre I had my fingers and toes crossed hoping for the best result. A couple of hours later I was woken up by a nurse in the recovery room. I was so sleepy and sore but after a short while I was taken back to my room where Matthew and my Mam were waiting for me. I could see chicken salad sandwiches and a cup of tea ready for me and I couldn't wait to have a drink. More nurses came in and out to check on me and check my drainage and everything seemed fine until Dr M came into see me. He wanted to have a look at my belly and check my drainage himself but by this time my belly had swollen quite a lot. It looked like I had a rugby ball underneath my skin and the doctor was very concerned. Suddenly I was rushed back to theatre because my belly was filling up with blood. I had to have my scar reopened and I was still awake while he did it because I had only local anaesthetic. That felt so strange. Dr M worked very quickly and he stopped the bleeding but the whole operation took about an hour and a half and because the time seemed to pass very slowly it felt like it was longer. Eventually I got back to my room and by that time I was very tired. I sent Matthew and my Mam home, it was so late and I could see they were tired too.

I had my own nurse who looked after me very well, but even though I felt exhausted I couldn't sleep and I was awake for most of the night. I was so glad to see morning come especially as I was allowed to go home that day. Dr M came to see me before I left to see how I was doing. He was very apologetic about the bleed but I said it was fine, just one of those things and that things do happen out of the doctor's control and it can't be helped. My mother came to get me. Matthew couldn't come because he had to go back to work. I had another appointment for two weeks time to see Dr M so that he could see how I was healing. He had already told me that if the operation had been a success I would know around six weeks after the operation and the first two weeks flew by so fast before I knew it I was back at the hospital. Dr M said that I was healing very well. I was still sore and I couldn't move around a lot but he said that he was very pleased and that I should make an appointment to see him again in a month's time. That meant of course that by the time I went back it would be just over six weeks since the operation.

The next few weeks passed more slowly and my pain didn't seem to be getting much better despite the operation. I wasn't feeling any real benefits and by the time I went back to see Dr M a month later there was no change. The operation hadn't worked and I was so disappointed. I could see Dr M was too but I told him at least I can say he tried. I was grateful for that.

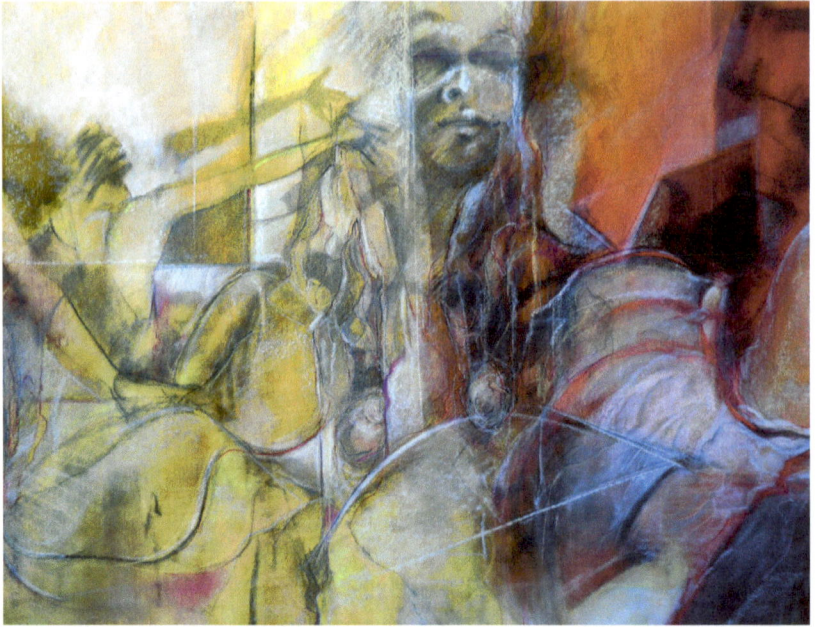

TRANSIENCE (DETAIL): *oil paint, chalk, charcoal, ink on canvas with oil ground*

This piece is a detail of a larger drawing (3 × 1.5 metres) which represents the whole of the *Drawing Women's Cancer* project. Imagery is here combined with textual content taken from transcripts of conversations I had with women and medical staff.

For they breathe truth that breathe their words in pain.

Shakespeare, *Richard II* 2.1

Pain

In basic terms, when we talk about physical pain we are referring to the way in which our body's nervous system reacts to the fact that damage has occurred, or is indeed occurring, to our bodily tissues. Physical pain is therefore a form of bodily sensation, a feeling of physical unease or disturbance that can escalate from a minor irritation to total and overwhelming agony.

Physical pain can be categorised as either acute or chronic. Acute pain is identified by its sudden onset, by its derivation from a specific disease or injury, and by its being self-limiting. Acute pain can also have a useful biological role. For example, the pain caused by placing your finger in a flame is enough to make you quickly withdraw your hand. In contrast, chronic pain is without definable limitation and persists long after the normal healing period that may be associated with a particular disease or injury. Chronic pain serves no biological purpose and, as such, can be itself considered a disease state.

Along with the division between acute and chronic forms of pain there are also two basic categories of pain sensation: somatic and visceral. Somatic pain occurs when pain receptors in bodily tissues, such as skin, muscles and bones, are stimulated by outside forces such as pressure, trauma, temperature, vibration and inflammation. Somatic pain can be further subdivided into superficial and deep pain. Superficial pain occurs primarily in the surface tissues of the skin and mucous membranes. It gives rise to sharp, pricking or cutting sensation and soreness. Deep somatic pain is identified more by an aching feeling because it derives from internal structures including tendons, joints, bones and muscles.

Somatic pain is usually localised to a specific area, although it can spread outwards, depending on the extent of the injury, across larger areas of the body. Either way, somatic pain can be erratic or constant and it is usually exacerbated by movement. Visceral pain on the other hand derives from damaged or injured internal organs and tissues and causes sensations of deep aching,

How to cite this book chapter:
Saorsa, J. with Phillips, R. 2019. *Like Any Other Woman: The Lived Experience of Gynaecological Cancer.* Pp. 157–159. Cardiff: Cardiff University Press.
DOI: https://doi.org/10.18573/book2.z. License: CC-BY-NC-ND 4.0

cramping or pressure. Unlike somatic pain, visceral pain cannot be accurately localised or clearly defined. It is diffuse and not well understood and it is therefore more difficult to manage.

But of course pain is not only physical. Emotional pain is often of equal stature in terms of levels of suffering and it is often not possible, or even advisable, to fully separate the physical from the emotional, especially where the painful condition is chronic.

> To be honest I felt worse after this operation than after any of them and after a few weeks I began to feel this horrible pain in my belly. I didn't know what it was and as time went by the pain got worse it was frightening me.

Pain is clearly a very complex thing, so much so that ways of understanding and managing it, including concepts of the meaning of pain itself, are different and perhaps infinitely varied among individuals. On reading Becky's narrative as it continues chronologically, and while writing up the transcripts of our conversations, it became clear to me that her way of describing the chronic pain she was experiencing, and indeed continues to experience, slowly and quite subtly changed over time. From initially being something outside of herself but which nevertheless impacted in a very negative way on her life, she began to recognise it as something that was actually part of her.

> The difficult part of all this is my pain. It is so badly getting in the way of everything, especially trying for a baby, and it's stopping me from doing a lot of things and sometimes it feels like its only getting worse. Some days I feel like I just can't bear it, and I can't find the words to describe how bad it feels except that it's like going through hell.

This was an interesting shift in her understanding of her own situation and it was manifest in the way in which she often struggled to manage her emotions when talking about the pain and how she managed it.

> I was feeling excited to see the doctor and I was hoping that he could shed some light on what was going on with my pain.

So, chronic pain, ubiquitous in its character and increasingly debilitating in its effect, slowly and subtly became a focus, a point of reference to which Becky's very sense of self was orientated, and her perceived level of control over it diminished just as surely as did her confidence in the medical professionals as they struggled to find the cause.

> For months on end not a single week has passed where I haven't visited a hospital but for all the examinations and tests my pain is still there.

Her language became more personal. She began to refer to the pain not as a discrete phenomenon, 'it', that she suffered from, but as 'mine', something that she owned, something that belonged specifically to her. 'It is my pain.'

> The next few weeks passed more slowly and my pain didn't seem to be getting much better despite the operation. I wasn't feeling any real benefits and by the time I went back to see Dr M a month later there was no change. The operation hadn't worked and I was so disappointed.

This form of psychological ownership is a very complex state of self-awareness that inevitably influences an emotional understanding of what it actually means to be a 'Self'. For Becky, 'her' pain came to be a vital part of the person that she now recognises *as* herself. The Becky who, before her illness, lived a busy and fulfilling life while working hard at the hairdressing salon is now living with a chronic condition that imposes limitations on her way of being that were not there before. She is unable to continue with her job because of the pain and, as such, the pain has informed a particular construction (or reconstruction) of her own self-identity, a fusion of her persona with the one point of reference that is at least relatable in its continued presence, even if it is not understandable. The pain itself and Becky's identification with it through a sense of ownership gives rise then to a new self-understanding, a new self-identity, which gives meaning to her life as it now is and allows her to manage her situation in as positive a way as possible.

> I'm also in the middle of having this treatment on my bladder to try and help with my bladder pain the nerve damage is all around that area my bladder is very painful and I feel I need to wee all the time the treatment does seem to be easing it slightly for me so that's a little help.

The question is not how to get cured, but how to live.

Joseph Conrad

The Aftermath

It is 2018 and I have reached the age of thirty-two. I don't know where the last seven years have gone. I realise now that when people used to say to me that as you get older the years go by much quicker, by God they were right. I am at the point in my life where me and Matthew are ready for a family. After the miscarriage it has taken a long time for me to get over losing my twins. I don't think I ever will really but I have to put it to the back of my mind because now we are ready to have a little one and just thinking about it makes me feel so excited. The difficult part of all this is my pain. It is so badly getting in the way of everything, especially trying for a baby, and it's stopping me from doing a lot of things and sometimes it feels like its only getting worse. Some days I feel like I just can't bear it, and I can't find the words to describe how bad it feels except that it's like going through hell.

Despite everything me and Matthew are looking forward to the future and I'm still excited about what is to come, and know that I need to accept my pain because this is how life is going to be for me now. I don't want to moan, and I don't mean to sound ungrateful but I really am sick of the sight of hospitals because life at the moment does seem to be about hospitals and more hospitals and sometimes it seems that all I've got is appointment after appointment. For months on end not a single week has passed where I haven't visited a hospital but for all the examinations and tests my pain is still there. My walking is very poor and some days I have to go into a wheelchair. This is so difficult. I struggle to accept that I am like this because I am only thirty-two. I'm very limited to what I can do and this really upsets me so that some days I can't hold back tears.

I'm still the same person, or I try to be, however bad I'm feeling. I still do my hair and makeup and it makes me feel that little bit better. There's been countless times when I've bumped into people that I haven't seen for a while and the first thing they do is pay me a compliment, how well I look or

How to cite this book chapter:
Saorsa, J. with Phillips, R. 2019. *Like Any Other Woman: The Lived Experience of Gynaecological Cancer*. Pp. 161–162. Cardiff: Cardiff University Press.
DOI: https://doi.org/10.18573/book2.aa. License: CC-BY-NC-ND 4.0

how nice I look, but nobody sees what pain I'm in. The only ones who see it on a daily basis are Matthew and my Mam. A few weeks back I started seeing a lady doctor, Dr H, at Rookwood hospital in Cardiff. It's a place where they specialise in nerve damage but I didn't know what to expect. She was very nice and very good. The things she spoke to me about were very interesting. She wanted to give me an examination and she was very thorough, but like every other doctor has said she told me that I'm a very complicated patient and things are never straightforward with me.

I told her about the weakness on my left side that has been there for a long time. I noticed it back in 2011, a few months after I had my operation for the cancer. I had put it down to being so poorly but Dr H was interested in why I had the weakness on top of the nerve damage in my abdomen and she said it was obvious that both together they were causing the problems I was having with my back. We had a long chat about everything I had gone through, and we also discussed what we could do to try and make my body stronger and ready for me to carry a baby. I felt so much more positive because I really felt that she listened to me. Dr H decided then that she wanted me to have a brain scan. I was a bit lost because I couldn't understand why she was talking about a brain scan when it was pain in my body that was the problem, but she explained that there was a possibility that I may have had a mini stroke when I had my operation in 2010. It was a massive shock I really wasn't expecting that. The scan turned out to be OK though.

Suffering becomes beautiful when anyone bears great calamities with cheerfulness, not through insensibility but through greatness of mind.

Aristotle

SUTURE 8: Old Lady. Vulval Cancer

Acceptance

The following is taken from the direct and unedited transcript of an account of her illness experience gifted me by an 85-year-old lady. She and her story are the source of the drawing titled *Acceptance*.

Well, I had vaginal discomfort. Like an itchy situation, for quite some time. It wasn't until that famous actress, she had rectal cancer… it made me go to my doctor. And I had that condition I presume for about three years before I saw, and I asked for help. My doctor examined me and she said it's unusual what she could see. It looked like warts in the vulva and then I was referred here. I saw the surgeon and he examined me and his advice was that I had to have an operation and I agreed to that, obviously because of the situation I was suspecting, you know, what I had.

I had the operation under epidural, which was marvellous! The recovery was absolutely fantastic. I didn't feel anything. I didn't hear anything, and I think they must have put something in to calm me down. And I was then here for seven days because I was so swollen from the operation. The catheter they used for me, they wouldn't remove it because I couldn't pass urine.

Then I went home. I still had some bleed and apparently I did have a haematoma for which I received injections in my stomach. Painless. The after that the nurses came every day to clean me because apparently I had some infection there.

I haven't looked back ever since. I am glad that… well if I had left it any longer I probably would have developed cancer. I was told that there were pre-cancerous cells.

Well, the surgeon here didn't say it was cancer. He explained that there are three stages of cancer and he said I don't know where exactly it is

How to cite this book chapter:
Saorsa, J. with Phillips, R. 2019. *Like Any Other Woman: The Lived Experience of Gynaecological Cancer.* Pp. 165–167. Cardiff: Cardiff University Press.
DOI: https://doi.org/10.18573/book2.ab. License: CC-BY-NC-ND 4.0

with you but when we do the operation we test it and we'll let you know. When I came to see him as an outpatient a few weeks later he did tell me that it was pre-cancerous cells and that they will keep an eye on me, which they have. That was three years ago and it's all cleared. Well I feel all right now. It's just that I've got other health problems. I've got osteoporosis in my back. The vertebrae have gone. I've got blocked arteries in both legs thanks to smoking, and I still smoke. And… er… I've got some heart problems. But then I'm eighty-five.

It's funny. I'm a weird person. Anything that comes along I accept it with calmness. I never get over worried because… well, I believe in God. And I think that well, what's there to be, will be. I'm not a religious maniac or anything, but I say my prayers every night.

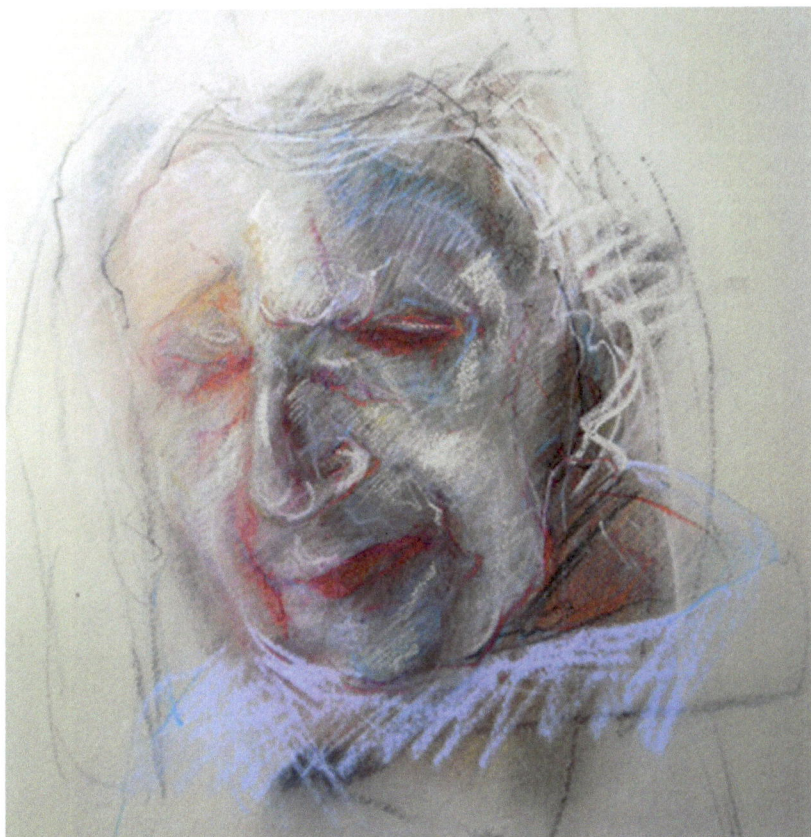

ACCEPTANCE: *chalk and pastel on paper*

This piece is inspired by my conversation with many ladies but one in particular, who accepted her condition with 'calmness'.

Becky. The BRCA Gene: Part 2

So much has gone on over the last few years and the saddest thing has been that my aunt became very ill again. The breast cancer returned and it was devastating for our family. She started her treatment straight away even though she knew how ill the chemotherapy would make her feel and her hair started going very thin again, which was really hard for her. But she bought herself a beautiful wig and even with all the treatment she was having she was still fighting strong. Whenever she went out she always looked beautiful, really smart and she never let her illness beat her. My Mam always told her how beautiful she looked and her husband would always pay her compliments. In the end the oncologist told her that there would come a time when there wouldn't be any more treatment and that was horrendous. Even though she was so brave you could see what it was doing to her inside and it was hard to watch. Me and my Mam would spend hours at her home just chatting and laughing and sometimes we cried. There wasn't a day went by when we didn't see her, even though some days I would be feeling really bad myself. We always made sure we went to see her. Her husband too looked after her in the best way possible. He did everything for her.

In November 2017 my aunt was very poorly and she had to go into a hospice so that they could control her pain. We all felt that she was in the best place, the nurses were lovely and it was like a very homely place. Her husband and her children didn't leave her side. Two days after my aunt went into the hospice my Mam was supposed to have an operation to remove her ovaries. She had chosen to have it done because she was carrying the BRCA gene. At the time though she didn't want to go through with it because she wanted to be with my aunt, but my aunt made her go, it was really important to her that Mam did it, that Mam would be less likely because of it to get cancer. A few days later my aunt passed away in her sleep.

How to cite this book chapter:
Saorsa, J. with Phillips, R. 2019. *Like Any Other Woman: The Lived Experience of Gynaecological Cancer.* Pp. 169–170. Cardiff: Cardiff University Press.
DOI: https://doi.org/10.18573/book2.ac. License: CC-BY-NC-ND 4.0

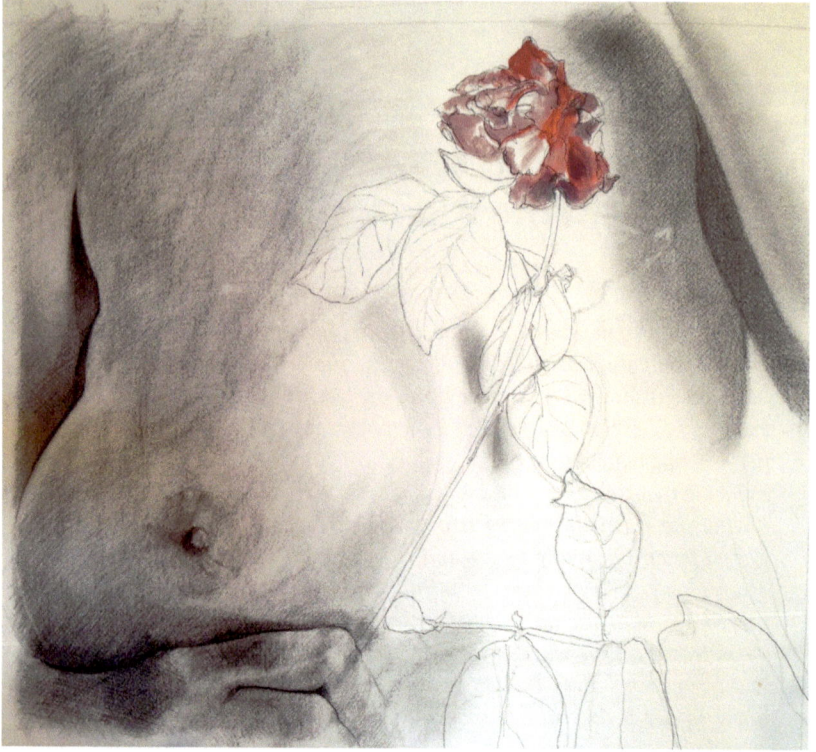

BRCA: *graphite and pastel on paper*

This piece is taken from a project about breast cancer, which in itself was a development of *Drawing Women's Cancer*. Originally inspired by the words and poetry of a woman patient who worked with me on this second project, the drawing is included here because I believe it also speaks eloquently to Becky's narrative. The crossover profoundly demonstrates how creativity and artistic empathy can transcend arbitrary distinctions in terms of human lived experience.

Becky. Final Chapter

I can't believe my luck I feel like one of the luckiest people on this earth! Let's take you back.

Because of my chronic pain we have been finding it difficult to get pregnant. It's not that I can't get pregnant; it's more of a timing issue. You need to have sex at the right time but that right time would always be when my pain was at it's worst, so I was getting quite stressed over it. I was thinking about it all the time. It was always there, pecking at my head. I was back and forth to hospitals most of the time and my gynaecologist doctors always knew that all we wanted was a baby. That was the most important thing to us. Matthew of course always needed me to be OK.

One of my gynaecologist doctors based at the Royal Glamorgan hospital decided to refer me to a fertility doctor just to give me a helping hand, and to me that sounded like a good plan. That doctor suggested to me about trying an IUI, which is artificial insemination, and I agreed to that and left the hospital that day feeling quite happy. I was looking forward to the future. I felt we were getting somewhere. It was just the waiting now, but I didn't wait long at all, only a few weeks, so before we knew it I had an appointment for the 15th March 2018. I was so excited.

Intrauterine insemination (IUI) is a fertility treatment that involves directly inserting sperm into a woman's womb. If a couple decides to have IUI using their own sperm, the man will be asked to provide a sperm sample at the fertility clinic by masturbating into a specimen cup. This usually happens on the same day that IUI treatment takes place. The sperm sample will be 'washed' and filtered to produce a concentrated sample of healthy sperm.

An instrument called a speculum is inserted into the woman's vagina to keep it open. A thin, flexible tube called a catheter is then placed inside the vagina and guided into the womb. The sperm sample is then

How to cite this book chapter:
Saorsa, J. with Phillips, R. 2019. *Like Any Other Woman: The Lived Experience of Gynaecological Cancer.* Pp. 171–174. Cardiff: Cardiff University Press.
DOI: https://doi.org/10.18573/book2.ad. License: CC-BY-NC-ND 4.0

passed through the catheter and into the womb. This process is mostly painless, although some women experience mild cramping for a short while. (NHS website)

Finally it was the morning of our appointment and even though it was a nice early one, we got there a bit earlier still. But that was my fault for being so keen! The doctor introduced himself and shook both of our hands so that put me at ease straight away, and he asked quite a lot of questions about my nerve damage and how it affects me. I explained to him as best as I could and I think he kind of understood but I really wasn't sure if he fully got how difficult it was for me. I really did try to explain how difficult sex was for me even at the right time and how sometimes I really wasn't well enough to do anything. All I needed was a little helping hand, but straight away he said IUI wasn't going to work! He kind of said that it was going to be a waste of time and he suggested IVF.

In vitro fertilisation (IVF) is one of several techniques available to help people with fertility problems have a baby. During IVF, an egg is removed from the woman's ovaries and fertilised with sperm in a laboratory. The fertilised egg, called an embryo, is then returned to the woman's womb to grow and develop. IVF can be carried out using your eggs and your partner's sperm, or eggs and sperm from donors. (NHS website)

Straight away I could feel myself getting upset. All sorts of thoughts were rushing through my head and I was thinking about all the medication you've got to take. I haven't been well for years now with my pain so I have taken a lot of medication over the years. It has been medication for this, medication for that, operation after operation and steroid injection after steroid injection. And then the timing was going through my head. How long were we going to have to wait? The doctor did say he would put me through as an emergency, so that meant it would probably take about six months.

I would go through fire and water to have a baby and so I kept saying to myself whatever the doctor suggests I will listen and take his advice. After all he is supposed to know what's best. But after my appointment, when me and Matthew sat in the car chatting about what had been said, I don't know why but I just burst into tears. I was so upset but Matthew put his arm around me and kissed me on my forehead. He said 'Everything is going to be OK. We will be fine,' and he made me feel better.

A few days later we went off for a week away in a caravan. It was a break and we both really needed it. We took our time getting there and had a nice ride. It did take a little longer than we thought because the snow was still on the ground and that delayed us slightly but eventually we got to the site and found our caravan. It was quite a posh one too, nice and clean and the heating worked very well, which was good because it was very cold outside. We settled in, and then we had to find somewhere nice to have something to eat. There were a good few nice pubs around. I was feeling very tired later that night and my pain was bad. I couldn't move around properly so in the end all I wanted to do was go to bed. The following day my pain wasn't any better but I wasn't letting it spoil our few days away so I relied on my wheelchair for the rest of the week.

When I'm in my chair I don't know why but people tend to stare a lot. I think it may be my age because I am still quite young and they are probably wondering what is wrong with me. In the end though, despite me not feeling very well we did have a very nice break and I think it done us the world of good.

I was expecting my period was during the week we were away but it was late. I didn't think too much about it though because my period had been all over the place for the last few months, Matthew wanted me to do a test but I didn't want to. I told him I wanted to leave it a few more days because I really didn't want more disappointment, but after a few more days had passed by and my period still hadn't come I asked my mother if she would pick me up a cheap test while she was out shopping.

Mam gave me the test as soon as she came back through the door and I done it straight away. I was so nervous. Well, I think everyone was! My heart felt like it was going to jump out of my chest as I waited the three minutes but when I looked at the test there were two lines showing up! One was very bright but the other was very faint. I could hardly see it but it was definitely there. I showed Matthew and my Mam and they could see a faint line, just like me, so we were all in the same state, none of us sure. I was still feeling very unwell with my pain so Matthew suggested that we jump in the car and go to get a more expensive test and that's what we did.

I waited in the car while Mam went and got me the Clear Blue test. Instead of lines Clear Blue actually says it on the screen, which is so much easier. When we got back to the house I had to do it straight away. My stomach was in knots and that three minute wait felt like a lifetime. When eventually I had the courage to have a look I honestly couldn't believe my eyes. I couldn't believe what I was reading because the test read that I was two to three weeks pregnant! The feeling that came over me was just amazing. I started crying. I couldn't control myself. It was the best feeling ever. Matthew and my Mam were just waiting for me to say something. They couldn't believe it either. We were all so excited. The one thing I did say was we have to keep this to ourselves until I had my twelve-week scan, and we all agreed. The only person I couldn't really keep it from was my best friend Lindsey, mostly because she was having a baby as well and we both share everything. We both haven't had it so easy so it was really nice to be able to tell her and when did she was so shocked and excited for us. Lindsey is four weeks ahead of me so our dates are very close together and two best friends having a baby together it just couldn't get any better.

I was so excited and nervous at the same time but also I was very impressed with how we managed to keep it to ourselves for those weeks. Mam did let it slip to one special person and that person was her sister, my aunt, Jill. Jill was one of the strongest people I have ever known. Just before she passed away she had a chat with all of us individually and the last thing she said to me was, 'You will have a baby Beck'. Them words stuck in my head and I think about her all the time. It was definitely Jill who gave us that little push we needed and it wonderfully, amazingly, worked! Mam visited the cemetery to tell Jill our news. I know that if she was still here she would have been over the moon for us. Mam misses her very much. We all miss her very much.

I am now thirty-two weeks pregnant with our little miracle who is a very precious little boy. We are so excited to meet him and we can't wait for either the 7th or the 14th November because that's when our miracle is going to be born by C-section. It's strange but so lovely that Jill's birthday is on the 7th November, but then I know that she's keeping a very close eye on me and looking after me. Me and my best friend are becoming first time mothers together and I couldn't have asked for anything more.

On 9 November 2018 I received a text from Becky:

Hi Jac,
Just letting you know that Reggie James Phillips was born yesterday at 9.28am. 6lbs 5oz.

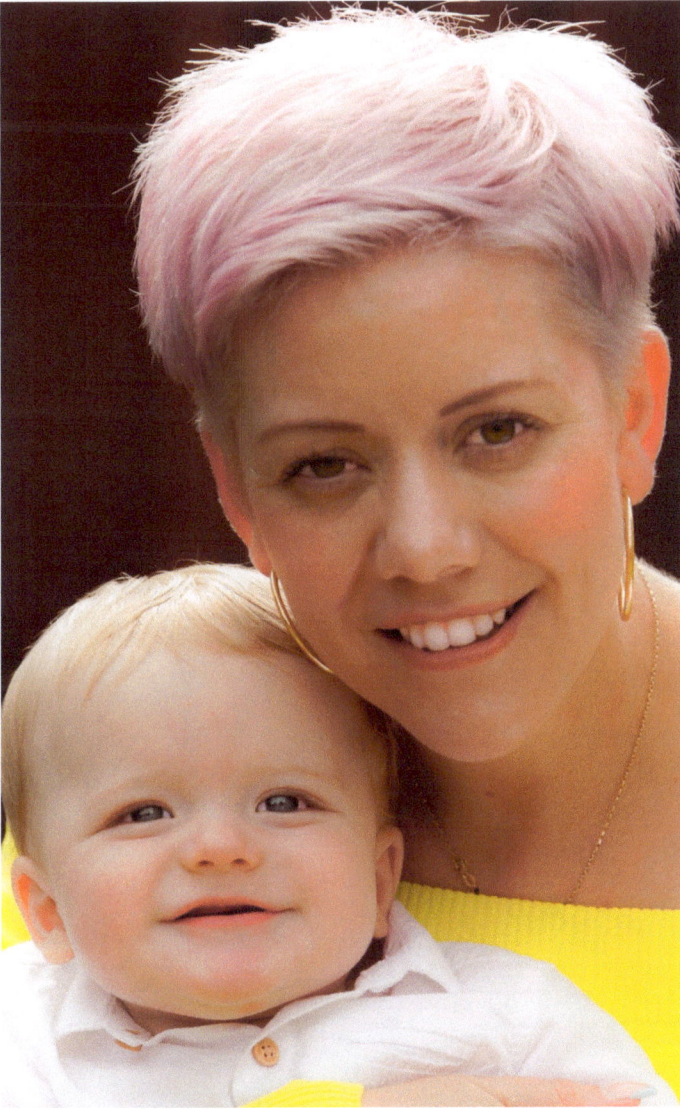

Becky and Reggie, July 2019

I have deliberately accredited Becky as an author in this book because although much of the writing is mine, it is her story, expressed here in her own words, that becomes the connecting thread that binds the whole. I am profoundly grateful for her courage, openness and generosity as she allowed me, through word and image, to share and articulate her experiences of the impact of cancer on a life. *Jac Saorsa, 2019*

This book is dedicated to all the women and their families, and all the medical professionals who gifted me their trust and their commitment to the Drawing Women's Cancer project.

Jac Saorsa
June 2019

This book is dedicated to my wonderful family who have supported me throughout, and especially to Matthew, my amazing husband, and Reggie, our perfect little miracle.

Rebecca Phillips
June 2019

A Chronology of Becky's Story

2006   Becky and Matthew, her husband-to-be, begin their relationship.

2007   Things start to get difficult with sexual relations. Becky begins to find it very painful when making love. She also notices a dark-coloured lump in her groin.

Becky makes an appointment with her GP about the difficulties she is having. When she attends she is seen by a nurse, who advises her that there is nothing to worry about regarding the lump and that she needs just to relax when having sex.

Christmas – Matthew proposes to Becky. A date is set: 25 September 2010.

Becky's beloved grandmother dies.

2008   27 September (Becky's birthday) – Becky and Matthew receive the keys to the house they have bought together.

Becky's smear test results show abnormalities.

2009   Becky and Matthew begin to plan their wedding.

Becky's second smear test results show abnormalities.

Becky undergoes a biopsy, followed by laser treatment to combat abnormal cells. During the treatment the doctor doesn't notice the unusual, dark-coloured lump that is still present in her groin.

At follow-up smear test appointment Becky shows the lump to the doctor, who, shocked that it is the first time he has seen it, takes a biopsy.

Becky contracts shingles.

Becky recovers but one 'shingle' remains and is suspicious. Becky sees her GP and is referred to a dermatologist.

2010   Results from the biopsy on the lump showed pre-cancerous cells. Becky undergoes an operation to have the dark-coloured lump removed and a second biopsy on the 'shingle'.

After the operation Becky and her family are told that there is a possibility that she has vulval cancer and that 'the necessary operation would be very disfiguring for a young woman of [Becky's] age'.

Becky receives cancer diagnosis: squamous carcinoma of the vulva.

Becky meets her oncologist and the plastic surgeon who will perform the operation to remove and reconstruct her vulva.

Date for operation set for 29 June. The actual operation is successful, however an accidental dural puncture causes a leakage of Becky's cerebrospinal fluid into her body and leaves her very ill in intensive care.

Becky is returned to theatre for a procedure involving the creation of an epidural blood patch, which effectively closes the puncture hole in her spinal cord.

Becky has a 10-day hospital stay during which she learns how to remove, clean and replace her colostomy bag.

Back at home, Becky continues making arrangements for her wedding.

Matthew helps Becky 'irrigate' her colostomy bag every morning for the two weeks before the wedding so that Becky would be able to enjoy her wedding day without worrying. On the day, 'I walked [up the aisle] very slowly but I did it. I could feel everyone's eyes on me but I focused on Matthew and when I got to him I could tell how much he liked my dress. He told me how beautiful I looked and that he wasn't expecting me to go for that kind of dress. He looked so smart and we were so proud.'

Becky and Matthew enjoy their honeymoon, a cruise in the Far East.

2011   Becky has more operations to take biopsies of surrounding skin.

The healing process is slightly delayed so Becky is told she has to wait to have the colostomy reversal operation.

2012   Finally, in the spring of 2012, Becky undergoes a colostomy reversal operation.

Becky begins to experience chronic pain in the area of the scar left by the colostomy reversal. It becomes so bad that it is terrifying and she begins a course of steroid injections along with various painkilling drugs.

Becky and I first meet, in the VIN Clinic at the beginning of the *Drawing Women's Cancer* project.

Becky undergoes an operation to lift the skin of her bottom around the original scar area. 'I noticed where they'd removed the skin from my bum area it had dropped. It was like... well, it was on the top of my legs so Dr D wanted to redo it. I wanted it done too. It was like having a bum lift!'

Becky starts to attend counselling sessions at a cancer care organisation.

November – The first public art exhibition for the *Drawing Women's Cancer* project, at the Senedd, the Welsh Assembly building, in Cardiff. Becky and her family attend.

2013   Becky and I meet for a second time. This time she invites me to her home.

2014   Becky's chronic pain continues and becomes debilitating. She is unable to return to work.

In the summer of 2014 Becky and Matthew are delighted and excited when she falls pregnant.

At nine weeks Becky has a routine scan. She finds out that she is carrying twins but, tragically, there are no heartbeats. Both foetuses are dead.

The aftermath is protracted, involving several further visits to the hospital.

Becky returns to counselling, where she has the opportunity to talk through her feelings.

2015   Becky tries to manage the chronic pain she is experiencing. There seems to be no answers as to its cause. Disillusioned with the NHS treatment, she seeks advice in the private health sector.

Private consultant advises that the pain is nerve-related and has its origin in the colostomy reversal. He advises Becky to see her GP and ask for a referral so that he can perform the operation that Becky needs through the NHS.

Becky finds out that NHS Wales has refused to fund the operation.

First doctor recommends another in Wales, however the waiting list is 18 months. Becky makes an appointment privately for two weeks' time.

Becky, her mother and her mother's sister take a test to show whether they carry the variant BRCA gene that greatly increases a woman's chances of getting breast cancer. Becky's aunt, who has already had breast cancer, finds that she does carry the gene, as do Becky's mother and Becky herself.

Becky attends an NHS appointment at Swansea Hospital with a team of doctors led by the consultant she had seen privately. She is told that the wait for an operation to try to relieve the chronic pain would be approximately three months.

Becky begins to suffer with painful symptoms that are like indigestion or heartburn. She is diagnosed with *H. pylori*, a bacterial infection of the stomach.

2016   Becky finds out that her name had been removed from the consultant's waiting list and that she is now on another doctor's list and the waiting time is indefinite.

Becky agrees to pay for the operation to be done privately by the original consultant.

The operation goes ahead but is unsuccessful. Becky's chronic pain continues.

2017   Becky's aunt, her mother's sister, dies from secondary breast cancer.

2018   Becky's chronic pain is increasingly debilitating and there seems not much that the NHS can offer her.

Becky and Matthew consider IUI and IVF fertility treatment. 'I would go through fire and water to have a baby and so I kept saying to myself whatever the doctor suggests I will listen and take his advice.'

Becky falls pregnant again – naturally!

8 November – Reggie James Phillips is born. A healthy 6lbs 5oz.

References

Aho, K (ed.) 2018 *Existential medicine: Essays on health and illness*. London: Rowman and Littlefield.

Bakhtin, M M 1981 *The dialogic imagination: Four essays*. Austin: University of Texas Press.

Boucher, G W 1994 The necessity of including the researcher in one's research. In: Tormey, R, Good, A and MacKeogh, C. *Postmethodology?* Dublin: Trinity College, pp. 11-20.

Charon, R 2006 *Narrative medicine: Honoring the stories of illness*. Oxford: OUP.

Coelho, P 2006 *The alchemist*. New York: Harper Collins.

Conrad, J 2004 *Lord Jim*. London: Penguin Classics.

Couser, G T 2004 *Vulnerable subjects, ethics and life writing*. New York: Cornell University Press.

Denzin, N K 2014 *Interpretive autoethnography*. London: SAGE.

Denzin, N K and Lincoln, Y S (eds.) 2001 *Handbook of qualitative research*. London: SAGE.

Frank, A W 1995 *The wounded storyteller: Body, illness and ethics*. Chicago: University of Chicago Press.

Gage, J 1999 *Colour and meaning: Art science and symbolism*. London: Thames and Hudson.

Hemingway, E 1984 *A farewell to arms*. London: Arrow Books.

Hippocrates 400BCE Aphorisms, 1994-2009. Available at http://classics.mit. edu//Hippocrates/aphorisms.html [Last accessed 14 August 2019]

Jarman, D 1993 *Chroma*. London: Vintage.

Kierkegaard, S 1983 The sickness unto death: A Christian psychological exposition for upbuilding and awakening. In: Kierkegaard, S. *Kierkegaard's Writings* (Vol. 19). Princeton: Princeton University Press.

Lawton, J 2000 *The dying process*. London: Routledge.

Mintz, S B 2015 *Hurt and pain: Literature and the suffering body*. London: Bloomsbury Academic.

Radley, A 2009 *Works of illness: Narrative picturing and the social response to serious disease*. London: Inkerman Press.

Saorsa, J 2012 Drawing women's cancer, 29 September 2012– . Available at https://drawingcancer.wordpress.com [Last accessed 4 September 2019].

Saorsa, J 2014 Medicine unmasked, 13 September 2014–25 June 2015. Available at https://medicineunmasked.wordpress.com/ [Last accessed 4 September 2019].

Saorsa, J 2014 Drawing out obstetric fistula, 30 October 2014–1 August 2017. Available at https://drawingof.wordpress.com [Last accessed 4 September 2019].

Saorsa, J 2016 Cancer Ward 12, 29 October 2016–4 June 2018. Available at https://cancerward12.wordpress.com/ [Last accessed 4 September 2019].

Selzer, R 1996 *Letters to a young doctor*. New York: Harcourt Brace.

Shakespeare, W 1595 *King Richard II*, 30th August 2008. *Available at* https://web. archive.org/web/20080830114449/http://etext.lib.virginia.edu/toc/modeng/public/MobRic2.html [Last accessed 14 August 2019]

Skloot, R 2010 *The Immortal Life of Henrietta Lacks*. London: Pan Books.

Solzhenitsyn, A 2003 *Cancer ward*. London: Vintage.

Sontag, S 1990 *Illness as metaphor and aids and its metaphors*. London: Penguin.

Sontag, S 2003 *Regarding the pain of others*. London: Penguin.

Sontag, S 2009 *The benefactor*. London: Penguin.

Speed, H 1913 *The practice and science of drawing*. London: Seeley, Service & Co.

Stacey, J 1997 *Teratologies: A cultural study of cancer*. London: Routledge.

Szczeklik, A 2007 *Catharsis: On the art of medicine*. London: University of Chicago Press.

Szczeklik, A 2012 *Kore*. Berkeley: Counterpoint Books.

Tempest Williams, T 2001 *Refuge*. New York: Vintage Books.

Tolkien, J R R 1995 *Lord of the rings*. Reprint ed. New York: Harper Collins.

www.ingramcontent.com/pod-product-compliance
Lightning Source LLC
Chambersburg PA
CBHW040126270326
41926CB00005B/90